FAT GIRLS
HIKING

FAT GIRLS HIKING

AN INCLUSIVE GUIDE TO
GETTING OUTDOORS
AT *ANY* SIZE OR ABILITY

SUMMER MICHAUD-SKOG

TIMBER PRESS
PORTLAND, OREGON

Published in 2022 by Timber Press, Inc.

The Haseltine Building

133 S.W. Second Avenue, Suite 450

Portland, Oregon 97204-3527

timberpress.com

Printed in China

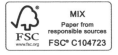

Text design by Lauren Michelle Smith

Cover illustration by Ariel Sinha

ISBN 978-1-64326-039-6

A catalog record for this book is available from the Library of Congress.

To my mama, Robin,

who made me who I am and taught me how to look
at the world through a camera lens.

To my sister, Sarah,

who always pushes me in the right direction
when I lose my compass.

To my besties, Ginamarie, Sarah, and Katie,

my rainbows, my ocean, my moss and moon sisters, your support,
laughter, and love mean the world to me.

To the Fat Girls Hiking community,

you have changed my life and made my dreams come true.

To every fat person

who was told they couldn't or shouldn't and did
it anyway, I'm proud of you.

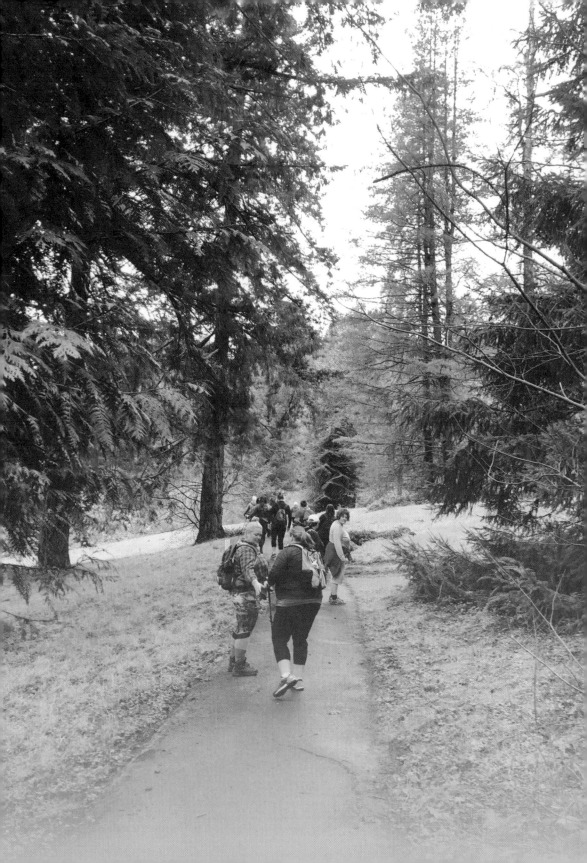

CONTENTS

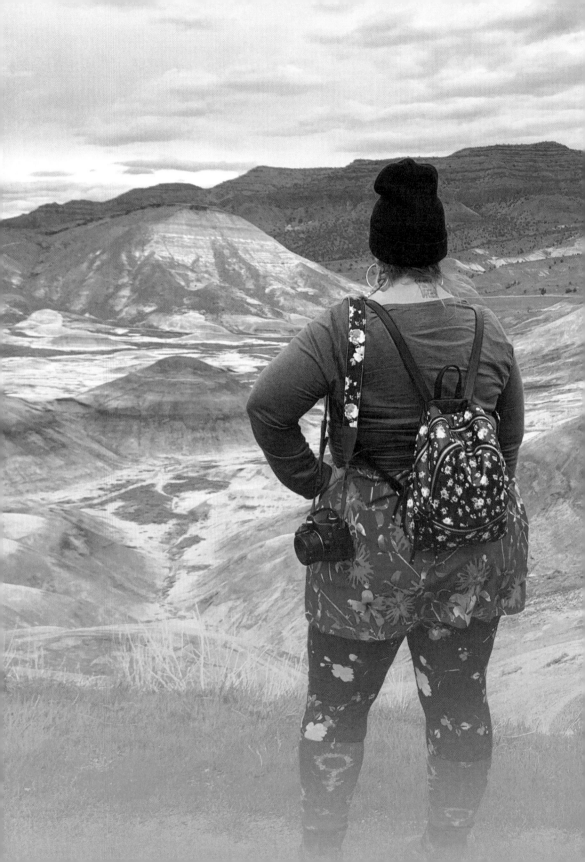

INTRODUCTION

In 2018, I traveled the country to open Fat Girls Hiking chapters, leading hikes and living in my mom's old minivan while also doing research. I had lead group hikes for years and found a glaring lack of information for accessible trails with inclusive information. Most outdoor guidebooks focus on thin, able-bodied hikers. I wanted a resource where folks with chronic pain or disabilities could find trails with benches, outdoor spaces that would accommodate mobility devices and wheelchairs, and specific information about whether bathrooms at a trailhead are gendered or gender neutral. These aspects of accessibility in the outdoors are often overlooked.

On my travels to open FGH chapters and find accessible trails, I would post in the FGH stories on Instagram about the great places and trails that I visited that center ADA accessibility. Shout-out to many of the national parks I visited! Many months after I returned to Oregon from my cross-country trip, I received an email from someone at Timber Press in Portland. They wanted to meet to talk about the book I was writing. *Ah, what book?* I thought. But as a lifelong writer, it was a dream opportunity. I had no idea how or what I was doing, but I sent in a book proposal and was honest about my mission. In that outline, I stated that I'm not an expert. I still don't feel like an expert—but my experiences and dedication to community, fat activism, and outdoor spaces that leave no one behind are valuable, despite what imposter syndrome tries to tell me. Needless to say, my idea to create a resource for outdoorsy people who rarely see themselves represented in the mainstream became my heart's work for the next fourteen months.

Most of this book was written outside at state park picnic tables, in my van, in small-town bars late at night, and, in the final push toward the deadline, in a yurt on the Oregon coast. I could not have written this book without the generous support of the FGH community, who shared the stories that now live in these pages. Trail reviews in this book focus on accessibility, and the reviewers' personal connection to the land. So many of the incredible FGH ambassadors contributed their favorite places in nature. Much of the work I do to keep the community a safer space for fat folks and all marginalized people is through my analytic work around cultural oppressive systems. Some stories I've written are funny, some evoke anger. As a writer, it is my job to tell the truth as I know it and examine all perspectives.

In 2020, not much was easy, and writing a book was no exception. As the world faced a deadly pandemic, quarantines, shut downs, police brutality, fascism from government leaders in the United States, wildfires on the West Coast, and ongoing environmental crises, it wasn't uncommon for me to find myself writing through tears. However, reading contributions for the community spotlights and trail reviews brought bright spots of joy into these days. The connections we all have made through online community and through group hikes and events have been so important to our collective joy. We are not alone!

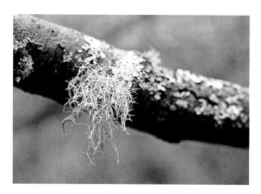

Moss and lichen are some of my favorite things to see outside

It's hard to know where to start with a new activity, especially if you don't see yourself represented in images of that world. When I started hiking, I didn't know it was something fat people did or could do. I hope this book will help you feel like there is, indeed, a place for you in the outdoors. You might be intimidated by certain gatekeepers in the outdoor industry—I was when I first started hiking, often feeling alienated by comments online or on trails about what it means to be a "real hiker." But I have also experienced a lot of kindness on trails. I have had some deep, soulful conversations with complete strangers in the wilderness—conversations I don't think are possible when I'm wearing my tough, city-girl protective shell. The outdoors makes me more open and vulnerable. At times it is uncomfortable. It's not easy to know where to start. But being out in nature is proven to make people happier.

I have learned through trial and error about the woes and rewards of getting out on a trail. Throughout this book, I'll cover all the little details that will allow you to feel comfortable as you begin hiking. What to wear, what to carry in your backpack, how to research a trail, how to find

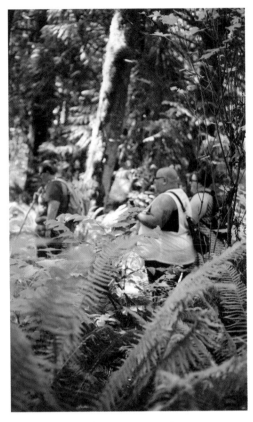

A group hike at Tryon Creek State Park in Portland, Oregon

ADA-accessible trails, and how to take care of yourself once you get there. The intent for this book is to spread the power and joy that comes from spending time on the trail. Along the way we'll celebrate who we are as a community, our individual stories and experiences, our collective desire for a more equitable world, and the incredible power the outdoors has to bring us all together. We all deserve to be heard, to see ourselves represented, and to have places that heal us.

HOW TO USE THIS BOOK

Fat Girls Hiking, the book, is a portal to different ways of connecting with the fat outdoor community. I assume that my proud mom will be the only one reading this from cover to cover. For everyone else, you can slip it into your backpack or display it on your coffee table and flip through it when curiosity calls or you need some daydream fodder. You might find yourself immersed in a personal essay from the FGH founder (that's me, hi) or really connecting to a community member's story.

The FGH community is full of people with lots of different identities and backgrounds who come together to support one another and find joy and healing in one another's company. This book shines a spotlight on some of these incredible people. Each member is finding their own ways to connect to the outdoors. Whether they're beginners or have been participating in outdoor recreation for a long time, their stories matter, and I'm so proud to be able to share them with you. I hope you'll also enjoy flipping through their amazing portraits and other photos—maybe you'll even mark some for future inspiration.

In my experience, outdoorsy people are always making new plans. If you're like me, your vacations probably center around those parts of nature you like best or where you've been wanting to hike. Do you have a hiking list? I love making them. When I first started hiking, before Fat Girls Hiking was even an idea, I had several lists for different areas of my state and other regions with hikes, campgrounds, and state and national parks I wanted to see. The lists were the seeds of dreams I planted and hoped would come true. Even just seeing photos online or in a library book would spark my imagination and begin drawing amazing adventures in my mind. Seeing some of those places in person has been a form of magic realized. If you want to start a list of your own, check out some of the trails reviewed by FGH ambassadors. There are twenty-six FGH chapters across the country, and each chapter has one to two ambassadors. They build fat-positive community, research, and lead hikes. I am so grateful to have their trail recommendations and incredible leadership. Their recommended trails are scattered all over the country so most won't be near where you live, but you can add them to your lists for places to travel to in the future. And they are a good sample of the kinds of trails that are out there.

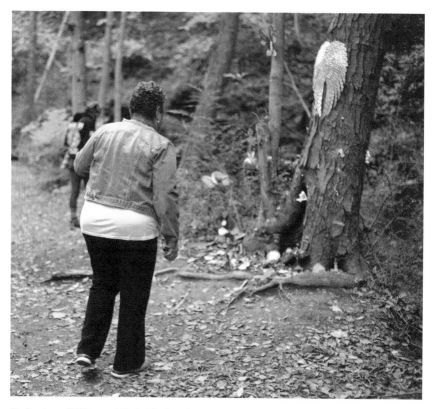

Trail art on a FGH group hike in Pittsburgh, Pennsylvania

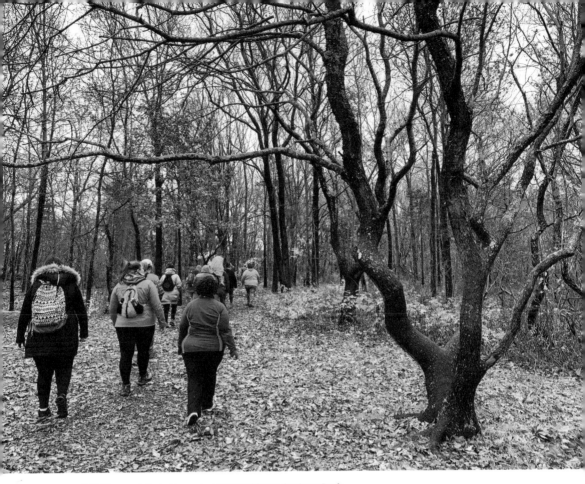

A FGH group hike in Massachusetts's Halibut Point State Park

Some trails hold personal history for the reviewer and some hold fond memories of a group hike—each contribution is a window into natural spaces that you can connect with as well. If a particular trail sounds like it's just your speed but it's thousands of miles away, you can use the characteristics the reviewer describes (like distance, elevation, or accessibility) to search for similar hikes closer to home.

Ever since I was a kid, I've always taken books with me wherever I go. Having something to read made me feel like I had a friend with me. I'm still like that. I live in a van, and my van is full of books. When I hike, I like to bring a book with me in my pack so when I stop for snacks or lunch, I can rest and read while taking in the nature around me. Nothing feels

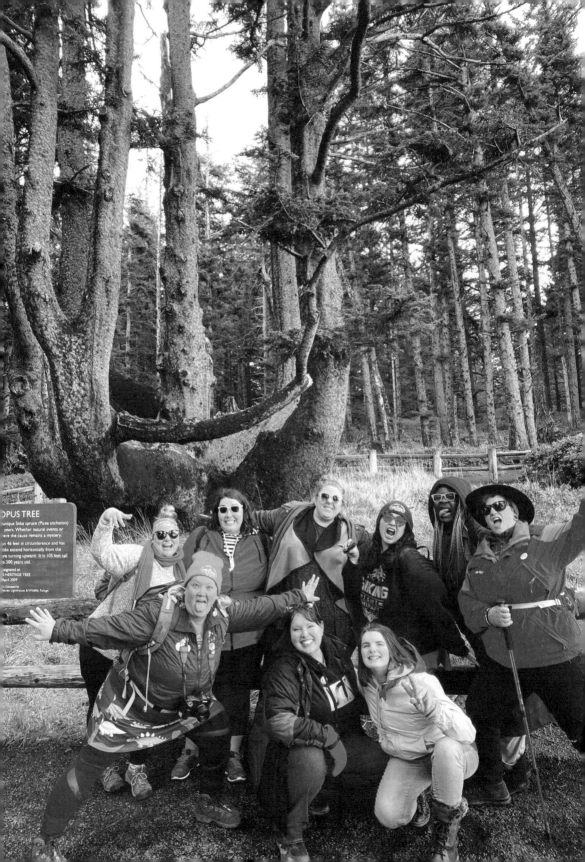

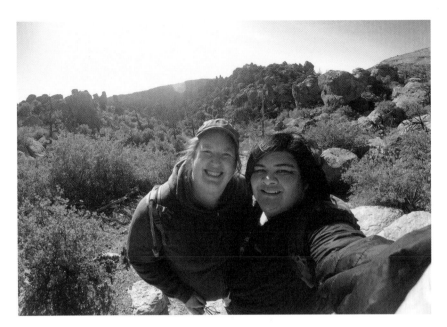

FGH ambassador Amy takes a selfie with her wife

more joyous than reading a book outside. This book was made to be hiked with and read outside in your backyard hammock or beside the ocean or wherever you spend time with nature. You can pick it up whenever you need to be reminded that you have a lovely community behind you, cheering you on as you spend time outdoors. However you spend time outdoors. No matter who you are. It's a reminder that you're not alone out there.

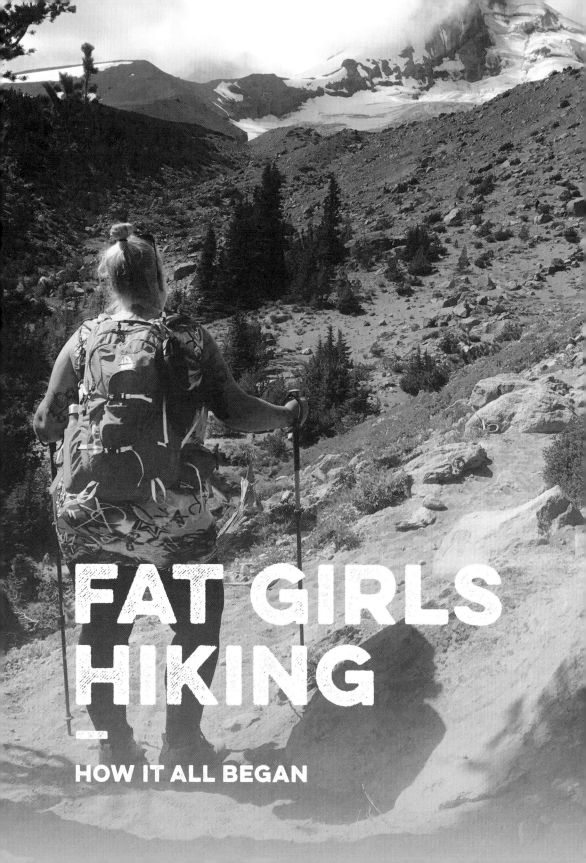

FAT GIRLS HIKING

HOW IT ALL BEGAN

n 2014, I was hiking a lot with my girlfriend at the time. We would make lists of places we wanted to road-trip to in Oregon, and I would research hikes and fun things to see and places to camp. After doing these sorts of trips awhile, I noticed that I didn't often see people who looked like me on trails or posting on Instagram about places in the outdoors. I am a queer, fat, heavily tattooed woman with chronic pain who hikes in dresses. I don't have money for "proper" outdoor gear and most of it doesn't even come in my size, so I get by with what is available.

Once my love of hiking and being outdoors set in, I scoured social media in the hope that I would find others like me. I did discover some online spaces specifically for women in the outdoors, but most typically showcased the same type of women over and over again—white, thin, cisgendered, heterosexual, able-bodied, conventionally attractive, and with all the expensive technical outdoor gear. There is absolutely nothing wrong about being any or all of these things, but I didn't see myself reflected in those spaces.

One day, I was on a popular trail near the Oregon coast with my girlfriend, and we felt like people were looking at us strangely—like we didn't belong there. Was it because we are a lesbian couple? Was it because we are both fat? Was it because I'm heavily tattooed and was wearing a colorful dress and she's Latina? We didn't know for sure, but it was clear that other people on the trail weren't used to seeing people that looked like us in the outdoors.

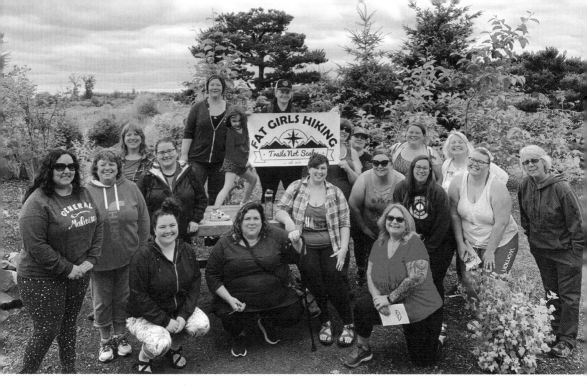

FGH group hike at Fernhill Wetlands in Forest Grove, Oregon

Often during our hikes, we would make up songs to pass the time or get through challenging sections. *We're just two fat girls hiking*, was the refrain that day on the Oregon coast. It made us laugh. It was a comfort to know that it didn't matter to us that we were fat girls hiking, we just loved being outside.

In 2015, my desire to see more diversity in outdoor social media inspired me to create an Instagram account called Fat Girls Hiking. I shared photographs and wrote about trails, campsites, and road trips. Though diversity in outdoor media, including social media, could be hard to find, some spaces had been carved out for marginalized groups. Some of the groups I looked up to as Fat Girls Hiking attracted a following included:

TRAIL DAMES A nationwide hiking club for "women of a curvy nature"

ESCAPING YOUR COMFORT ZONE An Australian club devoted to "body positive hiking and adventures for women and non-binary people"

SHE EXPLORES A podcast and blog about "inquisitive women in the outdoors and the stories, art, and connection that nature inspires"

OUTDOOR AFRO A nationwide network that "celebrates and inspires Black connections and leadership in nature"

LATINO OUTDOORS A community organization with a mission to "inspire, connect, and engage Latino communities in the outdoors"

MELANIN BASECAMP A blog working "to increase representation and opportunities for people of color in outdoor adventure sports"

I had been running the FGH Instagram account for a few months and noticed that other fat folks were using #fatgirlshiking as a hashtag. I wanted to amplify and showcase other fat women, queers, and women of color who were out here taking up space in the outdoors just like me and my friends. As I started to feature more people, the community grew. The more people I featured, the more it was clear that Fat Girls Hiking was no longer about what I personally was doing outside—it was a community that rallied around inclusivity, fat activism, and accessibility in the outdoors.

People began to ask for meet ups in person, group hikes, and group activities around this shared ideal. I remember thinking, *I'm not a hike leader. I don't know how to do that.* I was nervous that I didn't have the skills or experience to make an in-person community happen. But I started small, creating group hikes near where I lived at the time. The first group hike I posted on the Fat Girls Hiking page got a lot of attention online, but no one showed up for the hike in person. I did the hike anyway. The next two hikes, the same thing happened—lots of online support but no one showed up. I was disheartened by the effort I'd put in only for the "group" part of the hike to not happen. Maybe people didn't actually want to hike with me? But then, in June of 2016, five people showed up for a waterfall hike I planned. I was elated. Meeting people in real life who shared similar lived experiences as fat people was incredible!

Transitioning an online space where everyone is welcome to an IRL community space comes with challenges. On regular hikes with friends,

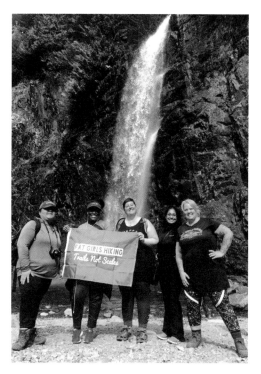

Because I had zero experience as an outdoor leader and was a new hiker myself, there were some early growing pains

we never talked about weight loss or diets, and we didn't shame ourselves or others for their abilities or body size. We also didn't use diet-culture language around food when we went out to eat after a hike. We would eat what we wanted and nourish ourselves in ways that feel good. There was no moral superiority with who was eating what and how much. I was determined to translate that same environment from my close circle of friends into a community setting, but I wasn't sure how.

When I started leading FGH group hikes, I was nervous to speak in front of a group, feeling much more comfortable with one-on-one conversations while on the trail. So I'd meet people at the trailheads, have them sign liability waivers, and we'd all start hiking. Because I wasn't clear about guidelines, sometimes people would join up without really understanding what Fat Girls Hiking was all about. As more people showed up with talk about their intentions to lose weight or excuses for why they were slow, I knew I needed to clarify our mission. It was a challenge, because I didn't want anyone to feel shamed for the choices they made for their own body, but I was trying to create an environment free from diet culture and talk. We weren't hiking to lose weight; we were creating a community where fat folks could be outdoors together.

Initially, I had described our group outings as Body Positive Hikes, but as the body positivity movement gained attention in mainstream media, the original intentions, meaning, and definition of that movement changed, causing people to misunderstand Fat Girls Hiking's mission and goals. I began using the phrase and tagline *Trails Not Scales* to emphasize the importance of a fat outdoor community that isn't focused on weight-loss or diet talk.

Online, I outright rejected diet culture. I spoke out against anti-fat rhetoric and fat shaming. And I stopped using the term *body positive* to describe our group hikes. I rewrote the mission statement:

Fat Girls Hiking is fat activism, body liberation, and outdoor community. We want to take the shame and stigma out of the word *fat* and empower it. Our motto, Trails Not Scales, focuses on self-care in the outdoors. We promote weight-neutrality and Health At Every Size. We want to create a space where fat and marginalized folks can come together in community to create safer spaces in the outdoors. Fat Girls Hiking is a community where people can access outdoor spaces in a way that meets their needs. We believe in representation for fat folks, folks of all ages, races, ethnicities, religions, classes, abilities, genders, and sexual identities. No diet talk, no weight-loss talk, no body shaming, and no bigotry of any kind is allowed in our online or real-life spaces. Our community is a safer space for marginalized folks and allies!

In addition to revising our mission statement, I started a new outdoor series called No Fatty Left Behind to promote greater inclusion and accessibility for our outdoor community. The name came from a fat-positive camp I attended on Orcas Island in Washington State with Wild Abundance Expeditions. The realization that some fat folks were unable to attend group hikes and events because of accessibility needs was heartbreaking for me. In bell hooks's book *Teaching Community: A Pedagogy of Hope*, she reminds us to always keep the most marginalized among us at the forefront of the community work we do. "To build community requires vigilant awareness of the work we must continually do to undermine all the socialization that leads us to behave in ways that perpetuate domination." This new series created room for folks in our community who need ADA-accessible trails, flat or no-elevation-gain trails, and places to sit along the way. It also welcomes folks who can't or don't want to hike at all but do want to spend time outdoors with a supportive group.

For our first outing of No Fatty Left Behind, a dear friend of mine agreed to give a talk to the group about their experiences in the outdoors. An optional, ADA-accessible hike followed the talk. We've kept this structure going as the workshop has evolved—these days I'll invite a community member with an interesting area of expertise to lead a workshop held in an accessible outdoor space. We've had workshops about body sovereignty, Indigenous relations to the land, plant identification, writing and journaling, and bird and wildlife viewing and identification. After the workshop, there is an opt-in walk on an ADA-accessible trail. This opt-in model accommodates the wide range of physical, emotional, and mental needs of the individuals in our group. It allows us to better focus on how we can celebrate and support one another in the community, challenging notions that we must "conquer" a trail or go a certain distance or speed in order to call what we are doing a hike. For folks who don't hike, we share an activity that centers our nature connection. Typically we will offer some journal prompts, reading material, or an arts-and-crafts project. We can sit near one another in the outdoors to talk about what it's like to navigate the world as fat people and explore ways to heal from oppression together, and this is enough to call ourselves outdoorsy.

I'm still nervous every time I lead a group hike. I still really don't like talking in front of groups. But I know now that other people see me as a leader, so I try to admit my fears and faults, evolve when needed, and face the community with honesty, vulnerability, and support. When people attend a group hike, I greet everyone (usually with a hug if they want one) and wait for people to arrive. Then, we make a circle so I can go over community guidelines and what to expect from the hike, giving each person permission to make the experience fit their physical, emotional, and mental needs. I tell them that we don't have a destination, that we can stop and turn around whenever we want to, that we are hiking to connect with one another, nature, and ourselves. Then we make introductions, in

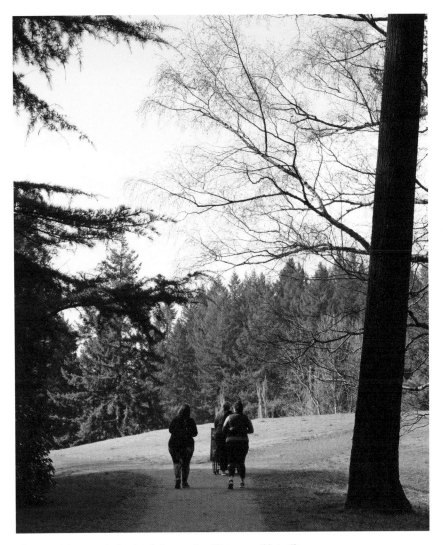

The Hoyt Arboretum in Portland, Oregon, has ADA-accessible trails

which I ask everyone to state their name, pronouns, and favorite thing or things in nature.

One of the biggest fears people have about joining a group hike is that they'll be too slow to keep up. Having been left behind on hikes by well-intended groups, partners, and friends, I understand this fear very

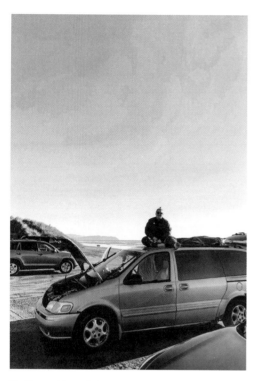

On the road in a minivan

well. Each time it happens I am filled with a feeling of shame, of not being good enough or worthy to be on the trail with people who are clearly more "in shape" than me. All the negative self-talk that society and diet culture feeds to me about why my fat body is wrong and bad rises to the surface.

To counter it, I remember that, at heart, I am still my teenage feminist riot grrrl self and she does not sub-scribe to toxic body ideology. Then I am gentle with myself and allow myself to celebrate my body just as it is at whatever pace it needs to go. When I slow down in the outdoors and go at a pace that feels good for me, I have an opportunity to catch my breath, take a lot of photos, and look around at the plants and trees. I'm able to appreciate and witness the beauty around and within me. I tell people on group hikes to honor their bodies' needs because I have learned to do that for myself.

Over the years, I have received countless messages, comments, and emails from people worried they are too slow and will hold the group back. I always let them know that no one is left behind on our group hikes and that we go at the pace of the slowest hiker. As the group leader, I am the last person on the trail. I try to ensure that folks in the back of the group, slower folks like me, feel the most support, because I don't want anyone to feel ashamed. Before we start the hike, I remind anybody who may take the lead to be mindful of where the group is and to keep a pace that allows people to catch up. This hasn't always been successful, but I set the intention. Sometimes people just want to go ahead and go faster than the pace of the slowest hiker. As long as the slowest hikers feel support from the group leader, I consider it a successful hike. Accessibility for the most marginalized among us is vital to creating a truly inclusive space.

Once I started sharing photos of our group hikes in the Portland area, people from all around the world started commenting. Things like, *I wish I had this where I live!* or, *How can I start a group like this?* I thought a lot about how to expand Fat Girls Hiking to other areas, but it was more uncharted territory. A dear friend from Knoxville, Tennessee, presented the perfect opportunity to expand. She'd been craving a community like Fat Girls Hiking locally, and after experiencing the FGH community on the first winter weekend retreat I hosted in Oregon, she was even more adamant about finding other fat folks in her area who wanted to spend time outside with her. I'd rented a house for the retreat in Mount Hood National Forest, and we cried together at the kitchen table, because we knew how powerful it was to be in a community with other fat people who weren't going to talk about weight loss and diets or body or food shame

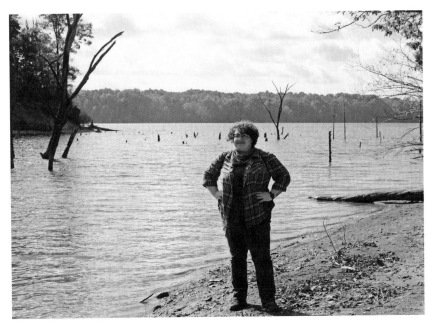

FGH Southwest Ohio ambassador Sara poses by the water

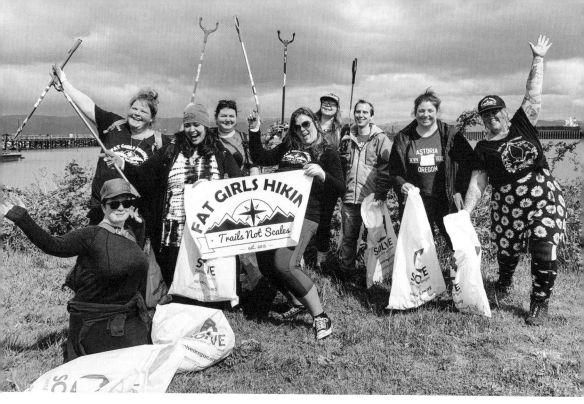

Clean-up hike in Oregon

themselves or others. Then we got to work creating the first FGH chapter outside Portland.

After I got the hang of setting up a chapter, I was excited to see where the organization would go. But I was also nervous about who the ambassadors would be. Would they understand the mission and uphold the values of the community? How would I explain to them how to lead a hike? I knew I'd have to let go of control and allow my precious baby to grow, but at first I really wanted to meet any potential ambassadors in person. This allowed me to get a sense of them, explain what would be expected of them as a group leader and ambassador, and ensure that they would uphold the safer-space guidelines. I traveled to Los Angeles; Seattle; Vancouver, British Columbia; and Minneapolis to host hikes and search for ambassadors. With their help, we created thriving communities in all those areas, where ambassadors host and lead group hikes once a month.

But the community wanted more chapters. So, I decided to take FGH on the road, traveling from Oregon to the Midwest and eastern United States to southeastern Canada. I lived in a minivan all along the way, leading group hikes, meeting amazing people, and eventually opening sixteen chapters.

But still the community asked for more. I had to admit it wasn't financially sustainable to travel everywhere that wanted a FGH chapter and meet every ambassador in person. So I created a questionnaire for potential ambassadors and emailed with anyone who was interested in setting up and leading a chapter in their area. If they seemed like a good fit, we would set up a time to talk on the phone. No matter how big the organization grows, I still want to personally ensure that every FGH leader has the tools to create an inclusive outdoor community that mirrors the one I started in Portland. There are now chapters all over the United States and Canada and even in England and Sweden.

The messages and comments I have received about my grassroots organization and community building encourage me. I am nurtured by the stories I hear on hikes.

Fat Girls Hiking saved me. Fat Girls Hiking changed my life.

I didn't know there were other fat people like me who hiked.

I'm so grateful this community exists.

People say they feel safe to be themselves in this community, or that they're inspired to take their first ever hike because of what they've seen online. The organization has changed immensely over the years, as have I. I hope we will all continue to grow and better ourselves. I know we will keep connecting online and in person when we're able to safely do so again. Fat Girls Hiking is the most challenging and rewarding work I have ever done. Thank you all for being here with me.

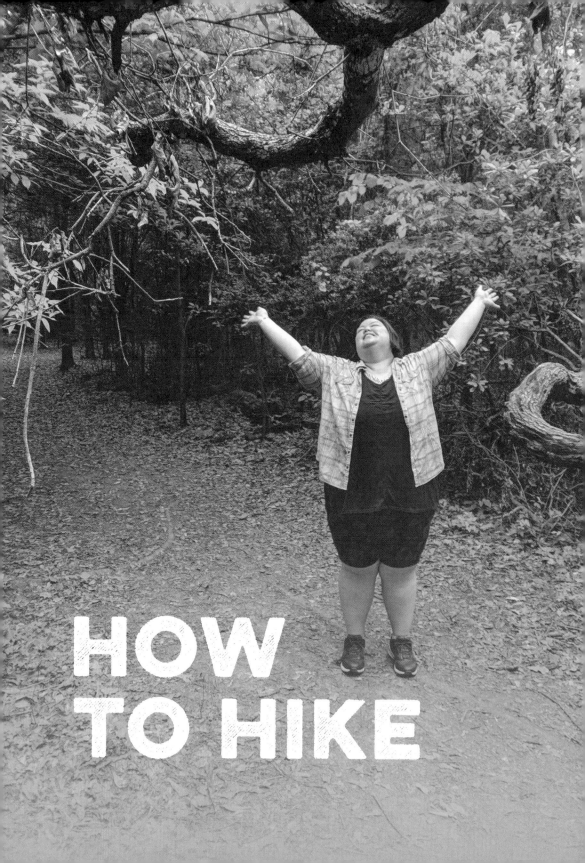

HOW
TO HIKE

WHAT TO WEAR

Listen, I like looking cute on a trail. I like feeling like myself, and I have a style that makes me feel comfortable and happy in my body. As a colorful femme who likes bright, sometimes clashing patterns, I haven't willingly worn pants in over a decade (leggings aren't pants, I've heard). When I first started hiking, I thought I had to dress a certain way to fit in or be accepted by the mainstream outdoor community. I feared that when I hiked in cotton or sneakers or cheap gear, people on the trail saw me as a fraud. But I didn't let the lack of cute outdoor gear in my size stop me. I hiked in leggings and dresses.

Eventually I learned why non-cotton apparel is so prevalent in hiking gear—it's much more comfortable when you get sweaty or wet from the rain. But I realized that my personal style didn't have to change. This was such a revelation! You can absolutely be yourself while hiking. Here's a list of things that have helped me find my happy place out on the trails in any weather.

MOISTURE-WICKING LAYER

Base layers (the clothes you wear closest to your skin) made of non-cotton materials are the best way to keep yourself dry. Most activewear—clothes intended for working out—works great, and there are lots of options at

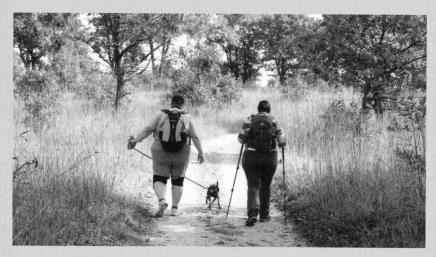

Hikers in northern Illinois

many price points. I like to support smaller brands and businesses whenever I can, but I know that they're not always financially accessible. When I first started, my favorite pair of leggings came from a big box store, cost less than twenty bucks, and lasted me for years of hikes. Now, my favorite hiking leggings have pockets (!!) that are perfect for easy access to my cell phone.

FOOTWEAR

The first hike I did after moving to Oregon, I didn't have any outdoor gear because I wasn't a regular hiker. For decades, the only footwear I owned were a pair of broken-in motorcycle boots. So I hiked in those. I quickly realized that they weren't super comfortable on trails (hell = rolled ankles), so I switched to some cheap sneakers I found at an outlet store.

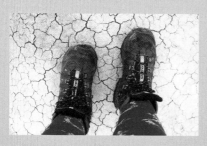

My hiking boots at Badlands National Park

If, when you're starting out, all you have are sneakers—wear those.

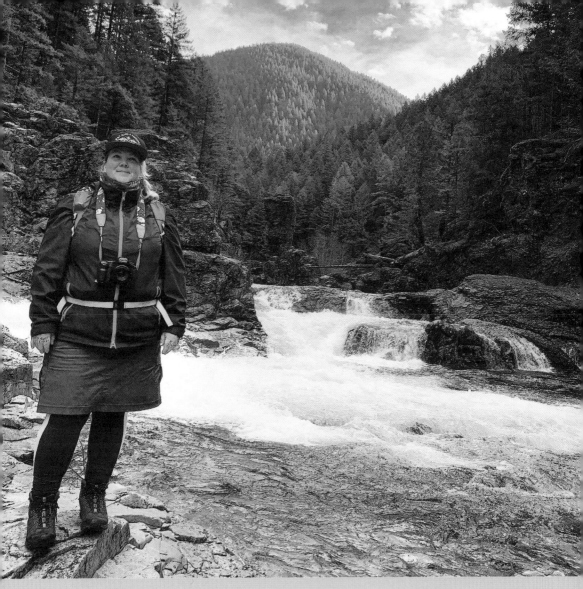

Rain gear is essential in the Pacific Northwest

If you live somewhere that's usually dry, sneakers may be the only hiking footwear you'll ever need. For me, sneakers worked better than my motorcycle boots, but I found myself with wet, cold feet on rainy days and muddy trails. Wet feet make me incredibly grumpy. If you're like me and you live somewhere where it rains a lot, you'll probably want shoes that can keep your feet dry instead of acting like wet, mud sponges. I find waterproof hiking boots essential to my happiness when hiking in the soggy Pacific Northwest. You can find waterproof footwear in more of a sneaker shape, but I prefer boots because I like the ankle support.

The final secret to comfortable feet is to have shoes to change into after your hike. I leave flip-flops or comfortable slip-on shoes in my vehicle for after-hike foot care. The sigh of happiness that comes from peeling sweaty socks off and slipping your feet into flip-flops is like none other.

WEATHER-PROTECTIVE APPAREL

Depending on where you live and the weather conditions where you'll be hiking, consider items to protect yourself from the elements. A rain jacket or poncho, waterproof pants or moisture-wicking leggings, a snow jacket and pants, or sun protection (whether it's a hat, sunglasses, or clothing with SPF protection) can all make your hike more enjoyable.

I know that finding technical outdoor gear is a challenge for people in plus-size bodies. The first rain jacket I used while hiking stopped at my waist—so while my torso and arms stayed dry, the entire bottom half of my

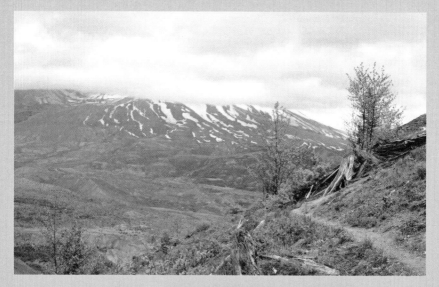

A cloudy day on Mount St. Helens's Loowit Trail

body did not. I suppose I could have worn rain pants, but, if you'll remember, I hate wearing pants, even ones that keep me dry. Because the outdoor gear industry is far behind in accommodating plus-size bodies, the solution so far has been a men's rain jacket from a big outdoor brand (it came with a removable puffer jacket liner that can be worn separately, which is nice). This jacket covers my butt, and that's what I wanted, however it's ill fitting everywhere else. In order to have a dry butt, I have to just deal with the baggy arms and hope that one day there will be rain jackets specifically designed for bodies like mine. I also dream about cute patterns and colors, but I'd take proper fit first.

HOW TO CHOOSE A BACKPACK

For me, a good-fitting backpack is an essential piece of gear. Everyone's dream backpack will be different, so research the fit, size, and features you want before you purchase. They can be expensive, but a quality backpack that you like makes a huge difference in your experience outdoors.

I bought my first outdoor backpack off the rack at an outdoor retailer. I was too intimidated to ask the people working at the store if it was the right size for me. In fact, I didn't even know at the time that backpacks came in different sizes and fits. Luckily, the pack I chose was mostly comfortable once I'd adjusted the straps to fit my body. But after actually using it outside, I quickly realized that some features would be really helpful for the weather where I hike—namely, after my first hike in the rain, everything

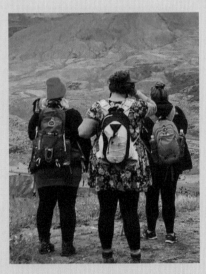

Besties at a favorite trail, Mount St. Helens National Monument

inside my pack got soaked. So I found a new, waterproof backpack, but, again, didn't ask for help finding my size. The straps on the new pack were uncomfortable, and I was constantly adjusting them to try to keep them from digging into my shoulders.

I knew I would have to spend a bit more money to get something that had the features I wanted and the comfort I needed—more importantly, I knew I'd have to talk to someone. Once I'd worked up the courage, I was able to ask an employee at the outdoor retailer to measure me for the correct size pack and let them know what I was looking for. I needed a pack for day hiking that would be padded on the straps and on the different parts where the pack touches my body. It also needed to be waterproof and have a spot for a hydration bladder, side pockets, and a hip belt for added stability. I was nervous that such a pack didn't exist for my fat body. It was no surprise to me that I had to shop in the men's section to find a pack with long enough straps. But in the end, I did find what I was looking for.

The best advice I can give about finding the right pack for you is "be brave." Talk to the employees at the store. I know it's intimidating. I know you feel like you don't belong there—in a lot of ways they are unwelcoming to fat people—but stand up for yourself as a consumer! You deserve outdoor gear that works for you.

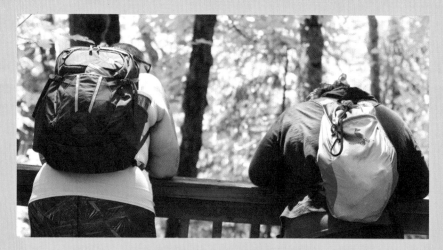

Daypacks come in a variety of sizes

FIT

Know that it is possible to find a back-pack with the right fit for you. Start by visiting any outdoor retailer (support small businesses if you can) to get measured. They'll measure the length of your torso from your neck to the top of your hipbone and can recommend packs in your range. Superfat folks may find that torso length doesn't provide enough information to find a pack that's comfortable around the arms and shoulders. It can help to ask people with a similar body size to yours which packs they like (online forums and communities are great for this) or just simply try on a lot of packs until

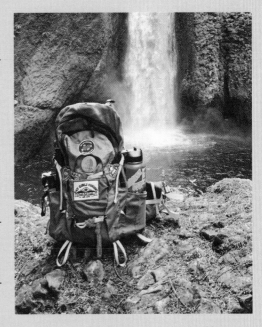

My pack at Wahclella Falls in Oregon's Columbia River Gorge

you find one that feels good. I tried three packs before I found one that was comfortable. Some packs have adjustable straps around the shoulders, arms, and torso, and playing around with looseness and tightness can help you find the perfect fit.

If you're looking for a pack with a hip belt (which provides extra support for heavy packs), you might have to get a belt extender, depending on your belly size. I have found men's packs to be more generous in their sizing. Even with the extenders, some packs may not work for everyone, but keep looking because your perfect pack is out there.

SIZE

It helps to have the right size backpack to meet your needs. Backpack sizes are measured in liters and reference the amount of space you'll have inside your pack. A pack listed as 16L means it can hold sixteen liters. If you are mostly going on day hikes, excursions that take half a day or less, a good backpack size would be between 20L and 35L. For longer hikes that may require bringing more food, water, and gear, your backpack should be bigger, between 50L and 60L. The daypack I use and love is 24L and gives me plenty of room for the essentials as well as an extra layer like a jacket.

FEATURES

Once you have a good idea about fit and know the size you want, start thinking about features. Backpack makers often include little flourishes that can be really great for helping you access what you need while hiking. Things like hip pockets aren't essential for hiking, but they sure are handy. I use mine to keep small items (lip balm, a hanky, my pocketknife, mace) easily accessible. They're also good for tucking away any little bits of trash.

My backpack has a zipper pouch on the bottom that holds a foldable a rain cover. This is perfect for hiking in the rainy Pacific Northwest. It also has a pouch inside for a hydration bladder that connects to a straw. I love being able to sip water without having to remove my pack.

PACK ESSENTIALS: WHAT TO BRING

The "ten essentials" for hiking can feel like an overwhelming list for anyone just starting out. Depending on where you hike, how long you'll be hiking, and if you'll have cell phone service or not, you may or may not need all these items for every hike. I'm a prepare-for-everything kind of person, but some of the items on the list I've rarely, if ever, used. In my many years of hiking with a well-stocked first aid kit, I've only ever used a Band-Aid and moleskin (for a blister when I was breaking in new boots). If you realize you enjoy hiking, you'll figure out over time what items you need and what items might not be necessary for every adventure outdoors.

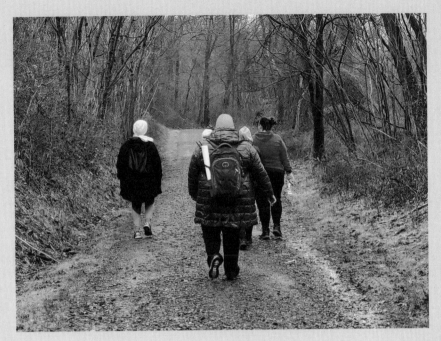

A group hike with FGH NYC

WATER

The commonly observed rule for day hikes is to carry one liter of water for every hour of hiking. However, water needs can vary depending on the person, weather conditions, and the difficulty of the hike—you may need to bring more or less water. Though it is heavy, it's always better to have more water than you need rather than less.

A hydration bladder with a straw is marvelously efficient. The bladders are light and don't create awkward bulges in your pack, and the straw makes it so you don't have to take your pack off every time you need a sip of water. Look for a bladder with a wide opening (similar to a plastic bag)—this feature makes it much easier to fully dry the container between hikes.

Being mindful of your hydration before and after a hike will improve your experience. Stay hydrated the day before and drink water on the way to the trailhead. Leave a gallon of water and a reusable water bottle in your vehicle so you can hydrate when you get back to the trailhead.

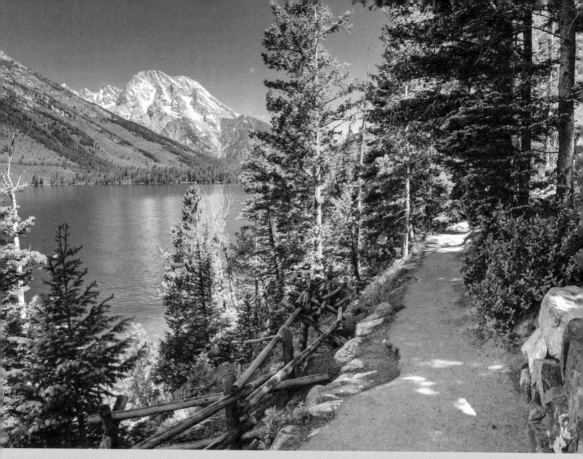

The ADA-accessible trail at Jenny Lake in Wyoming

FOOD AND SNACKS

Pack calorie-dense items. Protein bars, meat or tofu jerky, nuts, cheese, crackers, chips, cold noodle salad, candy, and sandwiches are great go-to food items. Always bring a little bit of extra food in case of an emergency. Some of my favorite trail snacks are peanut butter and jelly sandwiches, chips, Luna bars, and a trail mix with nuts, cranberries, chocolate, and sesame sticks. I've also been known to carry leftover pizza on hikes because there's something truly epic about chilling on a mountain and eating a slice of cold pizza. If I'm feeling fancy, I bring some sparkling water. A trail board can be fun too—sliced cheeses and meets with crackers and fruit. Get fancy with it. Pro tip: smoked cheeses don't mind being unrefrigerated awhile.

EMERGENCY ITEMS AND FIRST AID

Some things, like a water bottle or bladder, you'll use on every hike, others you might never use but should always pack just in case. I recommend keeping a whistle and a flashlight in your pack at all times. A whistle can help you attract attention if you need assistance and a flashlight (or headlamp) will keep you safe if you end up on a trail after dark. It's also a good idea to keep some sunscreen and bug spray in your pack in case you forget to apply before starting your hike.

A basic first aid kit should live in your daypack as well, so when you grab the pack, you know its got all the emergency items ready to go. There are inexpensive outdoor options available online or you can make your own in a waterproof container. Whichever you choose, your kit should include these items:

- pain and tummy medication
- bandages
- moleskin (a soft adhesive that's great for preventing and treating blisters)
- triple antibiotic ointment
- burn and bug ointment
- an emergency blanket (that can double as an emergency shelter)
- tampons or pads
- a how-to wilderness first aid guide
- stormproof matches
- (I also carry water purification tablets in my emergency pouch)

TRAIL MAP AND DIRECTIONS

Know where you're going and whether or not you'll have cell service. Some hiking apps allow you to download trail maps onto your phone so they're available if you don't have service. It's typically recommended that you don't rely solely on your phone for trail directions. I've had well-meaning strangers on the internet tell me that it's irresponsible to not have a backup map. *What if your phone dies or gets wet?* they worry. Well, if I'm hiking a heavily used trail with proper signage, or a trail I know well, or if I have cell phone service, I'm not as worried about having a secondary source for navigation.

The trails that are most accessible to me are typically in urban areas or are quite well traveled, so having a backup paper copy and compass (and knowledge of how to use it) isn't really necessary. If you're in an area you don't know well that also doesn't have cell service, or on a trail that isn't used much, a paper copy of the map and trail directions is a good idea. I'll be honest—I don't know how to use a compass. It's a skill I hope to learn one day but also one that I don't really need for the hikes I do.

I have only gotten "lost" on a trail once. Because I knew the area I'd be hiking in didn't have cell service, I had the printed trail directions with me. But, in person, the trails weren't well marked, and the directions were confusing and incorrect. I got turned around and wasn't sure where I was. It was scary, but I will say—I figured it out! And when I returned to my vehicle and consulted a second set of directions, it was so much clearer which path to take.

In all my time hiking, this kind of thing has only happened once. So know that it is unlikely, but still a possibility. Now when I'm on trails I don't know (especially if there's no cell service), I make sure to have multiple sources with directions in my pack.

The trail reviews in this book state whether or not a trail has cell service, and I think it's information that should be standard in guidebooks.

CAMERA OR PHONE

"Doing it for the 'gram" is a very real thing and there's no shame in it. I love to take selfies and photos of myself on the trail and to see photos of other fat folks outdoors. #representationmatters

I carry a lightweight tripod so I can get self-portraits in the places I'm hiking. When I take photos of my fat body doing an activity in which

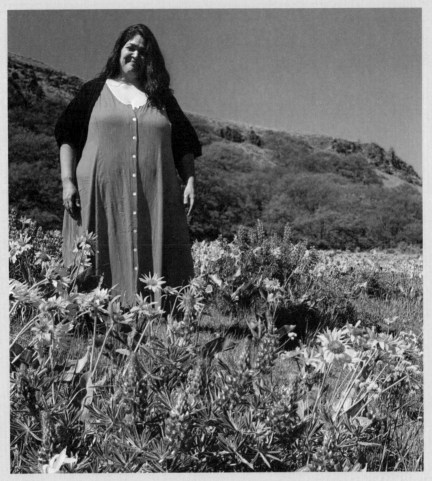

Ginamarie, our FGH Merch Queen, appreciates the beauty of lupine and balsam root wildflowers in the Columbia River Gorge

fat bodies aren't often represented, I'm celebrating what is possible for fat people. When I first started hiking, it felt subversive to be on top of a mountain, my belly showing through my form-fitting dress, my smile accentuating my double chin and expressing the pride I felt at having carried my body to the top of that mountain. I learned how to love myself more through posting photos that I used to deem "unflattering" because of how my body looked. It is truly revolutionary for others in fat bodies

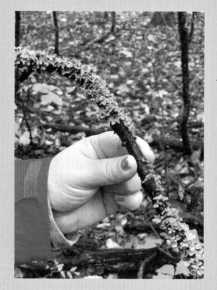

Investigate the small things in nature

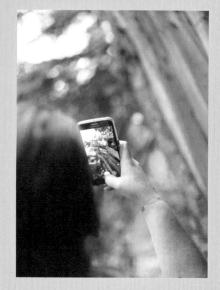

Take as many photos as you want

to see this type of media as well. So post those outdoor photos! Wherever you may be, however far you hike (or not), your body deserves to be celebrated and seen. You are allowed to take up space in the outdoors.

Having a camera is also great for taking photos of birds, plants, fungi, and moss specimens I don't recognize, so I can look them up later in my nature book. Identifying plants while hiking has become one of my favorite ways to connect with the world around me.

EXTRA CLOTHES

In case of an emergency, it's a great idea to bring extra clothes and moisture-wicking layers. You might not need that extra fleece, rain jacket, or pair of socks, but you'll be glad you packed them if you do. If you're hiking in rainy or snowy areas, don't forget things like rain pants, gloves, and a hat (I also bring a cozy fleece layer to add under my jacket if I get cold). For sunny hikes, I typically bring a cover-up with UV protection. If a hike has any creek, river, or water crossings, I like to bring my water sandals so I can keep my hiking boots and socks dry.

KNIFE OR MULTI-TOOL

There are many uses for a knife while hiking, from first aid to safety. I keep my multi-tool knife in my hip belt pouch for easy access—it has mini scissors, tweezers, a toothpick, knife, and mini saw. I've only ever used the knife—for cutting off a clothing tag—but I like having it with me just in case.

TREKKING POLES

If you're looking for extra lower-body support on the trail, I highly recommend trekking poles, those ski-pole lookalikes without the skis. Trekking poles help you step more confidently and with less impact, taking

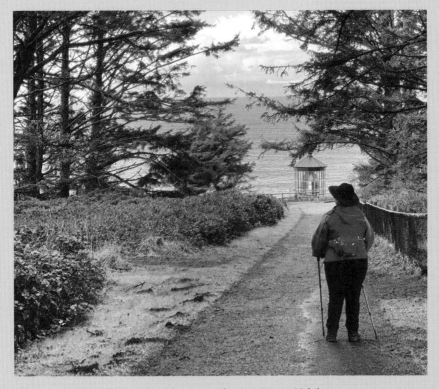

Erin using trekking poles to go down the steep trail to Cape Meares Lighthouse

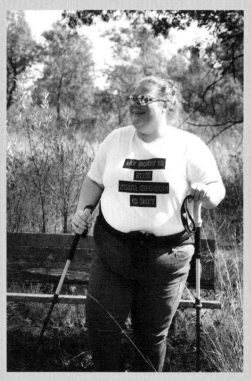

Lisa, who runs the Instagram account @plussizescuba, also enjoys hiking

some strain off your back and knees. My chronic back pain can make hiking a real challenge, and I also experience knee and foot pain when hiking up steep trails—I find poles alleviate back, knee, and foot pain during a hike and ensure I'm less sore after. When I have the support of trekking poles, I can navigate muddy or snowy patches more easily and safely, and on any sort of incline, up or down, having the poles is like having a railing to hold onto. I prefer telescoping poles that extend to different heights so I can adjust them as needed and pack them away more easily if I'm not using them. There are many different designs, in lightweight materials like carbon fiber and aluminum, and you'll find them at many price points.

FOLDING STOOL

When I'm tired on a hike, having a place to sit is a game changer. Camp stools are three-legged fold-up seats that can fit in most day packs. I always appreciate the rest and the opportunity to soak up nature comfortably. I have also seen some plastic stools online that are collapsible and lightweight with a high weight capacity. Don't be afraid to seek out and use tools like these to help you navigate the outdoors.

SAFETY WHILE HIKING

TELL SOMEONE WHERE AND WHEN YOU'RE HIKING

When hiking (alone or with others) in any area without cell service, I always text a family member or friend with the location where I'm hiking, screenshots of the trail map, where I plan to park, and when they can expect to get a text from me saying I've finished the hike. This isn't just good safety protocol—it also eases my anxiety and gives me immense comfort to know that someone knows where I am. Plus it's a great way for family and friends to support your hike from afar.

CHECK TRAIL REVIEWS ONLINE

I like to read user trail reviews on hikes I'm planning so I know what to expect for weather, trail conditions, wildlife sightings, and other relevant issues. Once, when hiking at Mount St. Helens National Monument, I read a trail review that a hiker had seen a cougar at the trailhead parking lot just a few days earlier. I was grateful to have that information so I could educate myself about what to do in case I encountered a cougar on the trail.

WILDLIFE SAFETY

The best way to stay safe in wilderness areas is to educate yourself on what wildlife you could encounter. I typically hike in areas with bears and cougars so I have researched what to do to prevent those encounters (make noise when hiking alone) and also what to do if an encounter happens. For cougars, don't turn your back, be loud, and slowly back away opening your jacket and spreading your arms to make yourself look big— fight back if necessary. For bears, I carry bear spray. Never approach or attempt to feed wildlife. Leave ample space between any animal you might see and yourself.

BE PREPARED

Make sure you have your pack essentials on every hike (even the short ones!). It's unlikely that you'll ever be injured or stranded on a trail, but if there's a worst-case scenario, you'll want to know what to do and have the supplies you'll need.

My first aid kit came with a small book that I keep in it on how to treat different ailments. Even though I've never had to use it, it's a comfort to know that if I was in a situation where I needed that information, I have it with me in my pack.

TURN AROUND BEFORE YOU'RE TIRED

Especially when you're a beginner, it can be tricky to figure out your limits. Do your best to stay in tune with your body cues. I typically know it's time to turn around if my feet get sore or I'm taking more breaks than usual. Some days my body can do eight miles, other days two, and some days no miles. When you turn around before you're tired, you will have a more enjoyable hike and limit the likelihood for injury from exhaustion.

There have been times when I've pushed past my tiredness to finish a hike or get to the destination. And while I did feel it was worth it at the time, not everyone is comfortable with that. It's always best to honor your own needs and speak up about them before a hike (if you're hiking with others) and during the hike. It's okay to not reach the intended destination. On every FGH group hike, I let folks know that while we might have an idea for our destination, it's not necessary that we reach it. Wherever we decide to end our hike is our destination. Group hikes are all about connections. We hike to connect with ourselves, with each other, and with nature.

KNOW YOUR LIMITS

Many mainstream outdoor information sources focus on how to finish a hike. Fat Girls Hiking has always focused on honoring the needs of your

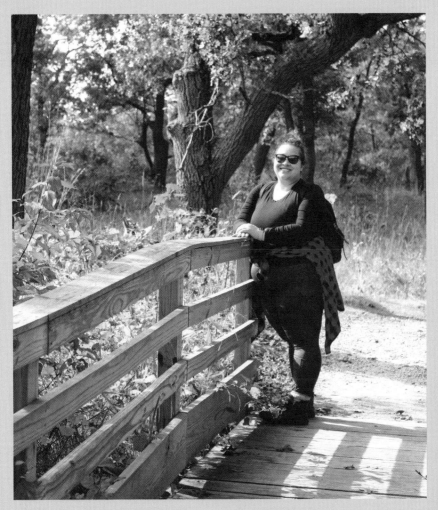

Have fun and be prepared

body. If you're new, and aren't sure how far you can hike, start by choosing short flat trails and gradually work your way up to more strenuous ones, if that's something you want to do. When you know your own limits, you will be able to enjoy the outdoors in a safer way. And give yourself permission to stop hiking and turn around whenever you want. The destination for any hike is the place you choose to turn around, not what a guidebook or trail map says. Be gentle with yourself if you don't make it as far as you expected. Focus on the joys of being outdoors and breathe the fresh air. No one decides how far or fast you hike except you.

HOW TO FIND A TRAIL

There is a lot of information online to help you find hiking trails. You can search your city (or any area) plus "best easy hikes" and find a lot of options to scroll through. If you want to narrow your options, you can search your area and filter the results by mileage, elevation gain, trail features (waterfall, lake, forest), wheelchair accessibility, and kid-friendly options.

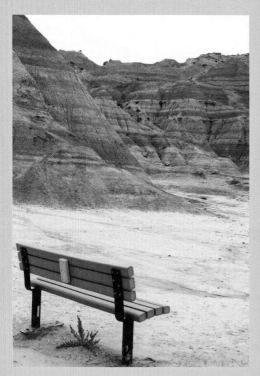

The ADA-accessible Window Trail in Badlands National Park

When I look for a hike, I consider the weather and what I feel like seeing that day. I live in the Pacific Northwest, which includes many kinds of landscapes—everything from beaches and rocky coasts to old-growth forests, rivers, high desert, mountains, and waterfalls. Think about what's available in your area that you might want to see and how the weather might impact you as you enjoy the outdoors.

MILEAGE AND ELEVATION GAIN

Mileage refers to the horizontal distance of a hike. Some hikes are out-and-back routes, meaning that you walk on the trail to the endpoint then turn around and walk back on the

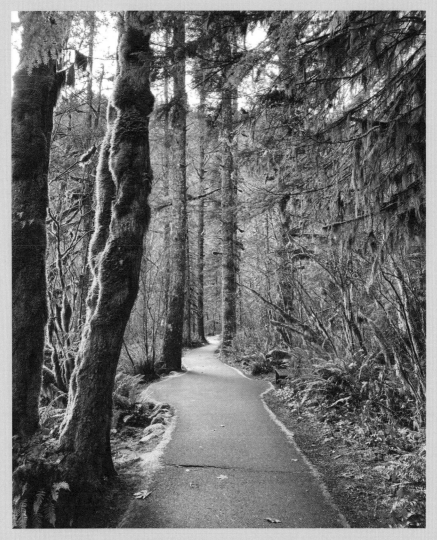

One of Wildwood Recreation Site's paved, ADA-accessible trails

same trail. Some hikes are loops—the trail starts at one point and loops back to the starting point so you're not retracing your steps. Some hikes are a mix of the two.

Elevation gain refers to the amount of vertical distance a trail covers. A good tip to consider is that 10 feet of elevation gain is approximately one

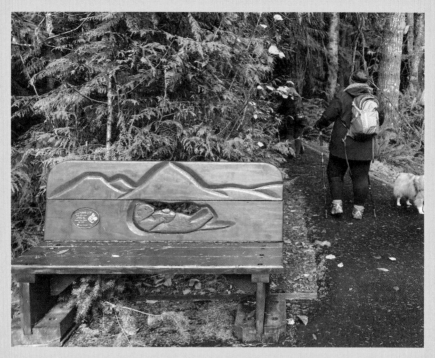

An ADA-accessible trail with carved-wood benches at the Wildwood Recreation Site

flight of stairs. So if a hike has an elevation gain of 100 feet, it's comparable to ten flights of stairs. Usually elevation gain is gradual. Most trails don't include stairs, but instead have switchbacks, which zigzag along an embankment so you end up walking farther but it's not as steep.

ADA-ACCESSIBLE TRAILS

ADA is an acronym for the Americans with Disabilities Act. ADA-accessible trails are considered pedestrian or multi-use trails that accommodate wheelchairs and mobility devices. Some of these trails may be paved or made up of crushed stone, packed dirt, or other materials. If you're unsure whether a trail is ADA accessible or not, consult online sources, call parks and ranger stations, or ask advice from folks in your communities (online and IRL) for more information.

In my experience, it's not always easy to find ADA-accessible trail info online. As a person with limited mobility and chronic pain, I have chosen to center accessibility in the FGH community. Ambassadors are asked to make every other hike they host (at minimum) an ADA-accessible one. I believe trails and the outdoors should be accessible to folks of all abilities. The number of wheelchair-accessible trails has been increasing, and I could not be happier about that.

Some folks may need a trail with benches along the way to sit and rest periodically. Many family-friendly hikes are now adding benches to trails to make them more accessible to more people. If you need to sit periodically, but the trail you're hiking doesn't have benches, you can also bring a small foldable camping stool to put in your backpack. Find the right tools for the needs of your body in the outdoors.

RESPECT THE LAND

One of the most important factors to consider when hiking is having respect for the land on which we recreate. We must honor and acknowledge the Indigenous people of the land, understand and follow practices that minimize our impact on the environments we hike through, and leave the land better than we found it by picking up and packing out any trash we see along the way.

NATIVE LAND ACKNOWLEDGMENT

Whenever I go hiking, I recognize that I'm a guest on stolen land. It's important to acknowledge when we are guests, settlers, or immigrants. All the lands where we recreate, live, and hike were stolen by white colonizers, and the deep histories of many lands' original stewards have been erased. Acknowledging the grave harm—genocide, deception, displacement—that has been done to Indigenous people across what we now call North America is the first step in honoring them. Educate yourself on the history of tribes in your area. What are the names? Do they still live on or near their homelands? How can you contribute to helping Indigenous communities heal? Where can you donate money to support them?

Native Land Digital, a Canadian nonprofit, has a wonderful website and app that allows you to look up almost any address in North America and find out whose land it's on. In addition, many local tribes maintain websites and are available if you want to reach out and inquire about ways to support them.

BATHROOM ETIQUETTE

Peeing and pooping outdoors is one of the least glamorous things about hiking. It's something folks rarely talk about but is important to consider before you go. When I first started hiking, the idea of pooping in the outdoors was mildly horrifying and not something I ever wanted to do. But nature calls when it calls.

As a fat hiker, I have found squatting to be tricky, so I like to find a downed log or a tree and lean my back against that for support while I squat. I also hike in dresses, so when I pull my leggings down, my dress covers me and maintains some privacy. I will admit to peeing on myself more times than I can count, but I will say that using the bathroom outdoors is a truly freeing experience once you get the hang of it and get over the lack of privacy and uncomfortable stance. Like most things, it just takes some practice. Try it in your yard a few times if you're really nervous about it.

The rules about where to relieve yourself can vary depending upon environmental factors, but, in general, keep these rules in mind: go at least 200 feet (about seventy adult paces) from water sources and trails, pack out your toilet paper, and bury your poop 6–8 inches deep (unless you're in an area that requires you to pack poop out as well). I have a big plastic bag in my backpack with a roll of toilet paper, wipes, hand sanitizer, and a trowel with measurements marking inches. Also, make sure you have some extra bags for the used toilet paper and wipes. In some environments, urine can attract wildlife. You can urinate on rocks, pine

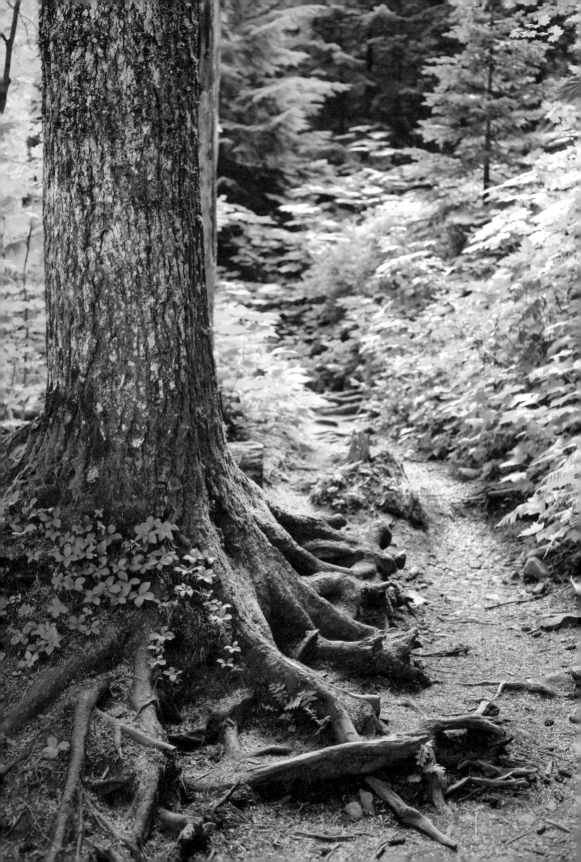

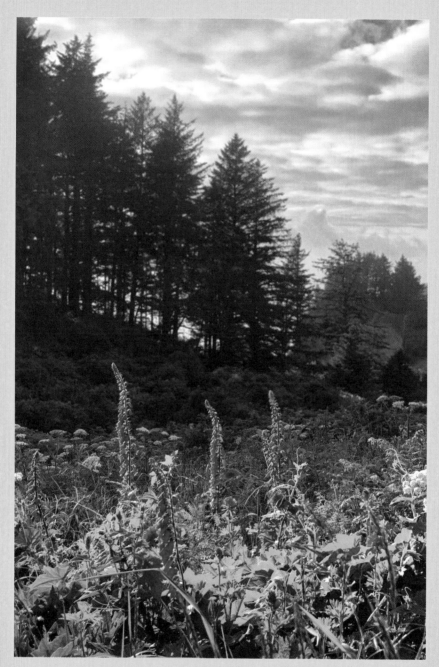

Foxgloves on Neahkahnie Mountain in summer

needles, or gravel and dilute your urine with a little water to minimize its impact on the environment.

MINIMIZE YOUR IMPACT

Remember to take care of the environment where you hike and minimize your impact on the land. You'll often see this described as Leave No Trace. We all need to do our part to keep natural areas beautiful for tomorrow's visitors and for future generations.

RESEARCH AND PLAN AHEAD Your hike or outdoor adventure should involve some planning to ensure a safe and enjoyable experience. Research the hike and area to make sure it meets your needs and capabilities. Know what rules and regulations may be in place (some areas have limits on group size or may not be accessible to folks without specific wilderness skills). Check weather reports to make sure you bring the proper gear and are mentally prepared for the conditions. Pack adequate food, water, and ways to dispose of your waste properly.

STAY ON TRAIL To minimize impact to natural areas, stay on designated trails. (There are times when you may need to go off trail to use "the bathroom" or take a break—in this case, be sure to follow best practices.)

WASTE DISPOSAL Pack it in, pack it out! Any trash you bring with you on a hike should return with you. This includes food scraps (including things like nut shells and fruit peels), paper products, and any other items you would throw away. I keep several small heavy-duty freezer bags in my pack for such items. Educate yourself on the guidelines for solid human waste in the area where you're hiking—some places allow it to be buried, others require you to pack it out (see the previous section for more guidelines on outdoor bathroom etiquette).

TAKE ONLY PHOTOS The best practice when in natural areas is to not pick wildflowers, damage trees (by carving or cutting them), move rocks, or take any natural items away from the spot where you find them—aka take only photos. However, I have been known to take home a mossy stick or two that's been blown down onto the trail by the wind. This rule doesn't necessarily take into account foraging and cultural connections people have to the land that may allow for exceptions, but it's a good place to start.

WILDLIFE SAFETY For your own safety and the safety of wildlife, please be considerate of your actions and their impacts. Keep your distance from wildlife. Educate yourself on what wildlife may be present in the area where you're hiking. Store food properly and don't feed wildlife.

OTHER PEOPLE Consider the choices you make and how they may impact others on the trail. Group size can considerably change another hiker's experience. There are some natural areas where group size is limited. Check what is suggested and split your group up if necessary. Avoid making a lot of noise or playing amplified music. Know and observe the protocol for sharing a narrow trail: downhill hikers should yield (step aside) to those hiking uphill—this keeps the flow of hikers moving.

SELF-CARE WHILE HIKING

HONOR THE NEEDS OF YOUR BODY

Take breaks. Take photos. Self-care is a huge component of the FGH community. We encourage breaks when you need them and going at the speed that feels good to you. "Go at your own pace" is literally one of our slogans. Give yourself permission to stop, turn around, or take a break whenever you need to—catch your breath, have some water, sit down, get a snack, or take some photos. The joy and healing I found in the outdoors came when I started really listening to my intuition. If something isn't feeling good, or feels too hard or unsafe, I stop. It can be a challenge

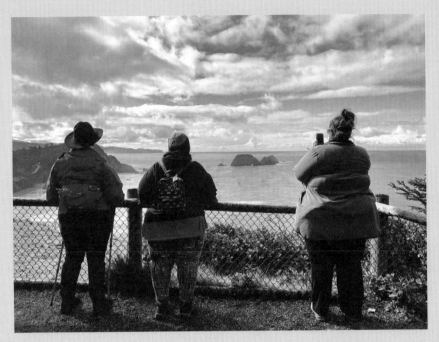

Take breaks to appreciate the view and to snap photos and selfies

to hear that inner voice at times, especially since we receive a lot of messages that tell us to follow the crowd or succeed at all costs.

I know shame can pop up at any moment when I practice joyful movement. New activities especially can be a real challenge. But not knowing how to do something is okay. It takes time and a lot of affirming self-talk to reframe our inner dialogue into something that benefits us. I still hear myself say things like, *I'm bad at rock climbing, why am I even doing this?* But with practice, I've learned to reframe that dialogue and talk back, saying, *You are trying something new and learning a skill you're not sure about. It's okay to feel apprehensive. It's okay to be bad at something. It's okay to fail. It's awesome that you are even doing this new activity! I'm proud of you.*

Sometimes anti-fat ideas I've heard that say I don't belong in the outdoors will float unbidden through my mind. Or I'll think of moments when someone made a comment about my abilities, my body, or just the

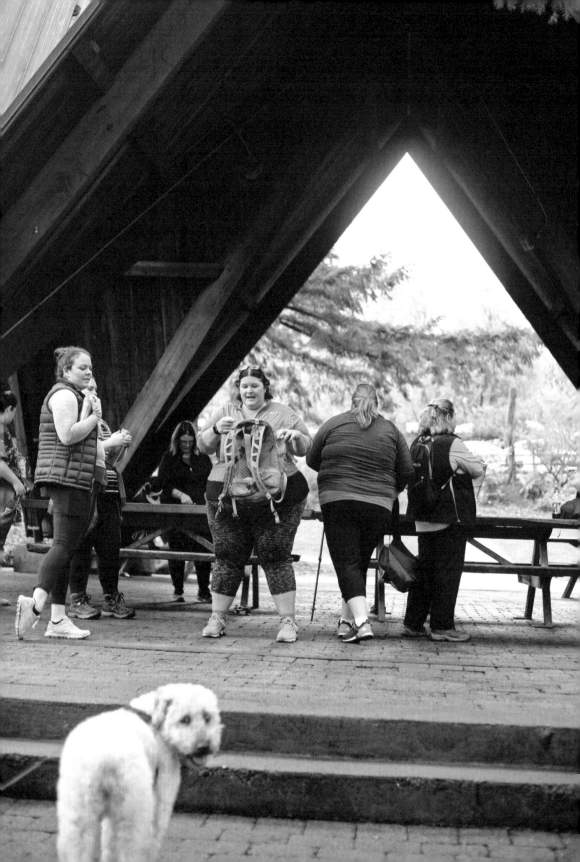

way I breathe when hiking. I remind myself that I am welcome to go anywhere I want and that other people's biases say more about them than me. I also remind myself that breathing heavy isn't shameful. My body does what it's supposed to when I'm working hard. I can stop as often as I want to catch my breath.

Self-care in the outdoors means I tell myself the story about me that I know to be true. I keep on listening to my inner voice. Eventually, it does become easier to hear.

Practice, that's all it takes. Do the thing. You will discover your inner voice and a strength you didn't know you had. You may cry, be in pain at times, or face scary situations, but you will persevere. Be kind to yourself. Give yourself the care you need. You deserve it. And you belong here.

AFTER-HIKE CARE

Spoil yourself.

I mean it. What do you need or want after a hike? Rest, hydration, food, and reflection. Eat some food you like, drink water, put on comfy clothes and shoes.

Ask yourself how you're feeling and take some ibuprofen or your preferred pain medicine if you need it. Allow yourself rest and reflection. I enjoy journaling about my experiences on the trail after hiking. And post those selfies, cuz I wanna see all you fat babes taking up space in the outdoors!

Whenever I lead a group hike, my favorite thing to do post-hike is share a meal with everybody. It's lovely to connect and refuel after being together on the trail. Before a hike, I'll often research cafes, diners, and restaurants in the area so that afterward we can support the local economy in those places. My favorite post-hike treat is a brewpub with a good burger and fries.

FINDING JOYFUL MOVEMENT

—

FITNESS TRAUMA, TEAM SPORTS, AND FAT ATHLETES

When I was in middle school in rural Minnesota, I loved track and field. But I was slow. Competitive sports aren't exactly the best place if you're slow like me. I enjoyed active group experiences, but the more I participated and was told that I wasn't "good" at the activity because I was slow or my body was bigger than others' my age, the more I told myself I just wasn't athletic. Somehow, even though I enjoyed gymnastics and dance as an adolescent, I could never be good at it because I was chubby. So I gave up. Teachers, instructors, and coaches didn't support me. When we took the presidential fitness test, the entire class would be changed out of their gym clothes and gossiping before I finished running the mile. It was easier for me to give up and say that sports weren't for me than to fight the system that kept telling me the way I looked and the way I performed would never be good enough. No one seems to care if you ran your personal best if you're the last in your class.

I stopped doing things I loved. They told me I should try harder and do better. I knew I was doing the best I could. I compared myself to others because that's what sports are designed for. I was seen as less than—shamed, bullied, and ridiculed—for not performing in the same ways as my peers. Nobody considered my individual abilities. This is the core root of my fitness trauma and why I stopped liking competitive team sports.

Gym class was my least favorite time at school. The group of girls who bullied me always amped up their criticism of my body in the locker room while we changed. I was teased for my style of underwear, my thicker

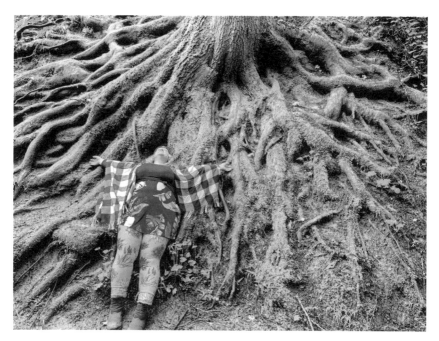

Connecting with nature can bring so much joy

thighs, my hair, my lack of trendy gym clothes. My attempts to hide my body under a towel while I changed made them laugh harder. After that, I always changed in the bathroom stalls.

Once we were in the gym or outside on the track out of ear range from adults, the comments continued. Anything I did was laughed at or criticized. If I made a mistake, I was wrong. If I did well, I was wrong. It seemed they hated me simply because I was fat and poor. These girls didn't really even know me, nor would I ever let them. Their bullying took a toll. I spent years in shame, thinking I was bad and wrong and should do anything I could to conform. I desperately wanted to fit in, to be accepted, and feel good having fun playing volleyball in the gymnasium.

The bullies I encountered at a young age had absorbed the messages of toxic diet culture, fat oppression, and weight bias. And they are sadly no different than the online trolls I now face in my work with Fat Girls Hiking. American society perpetuates the idea that fat people are less-than—that we are unintelligent, lazy, and incapable of the same physical feats as people in smaller bodies.

As a kid I thought, *gymnastics is for kids with parents that can afford private classes.* And, *track and field is for kids who are faster than me.* And, *dance is for kids with a certain body type.* These ideas didn't come from my parents but from instructors and coaches. These activities I loved and thought were fun gradually became a source of shame because I didn't fit the cultural standards of fitness. The trauma sank inside me, whispering, *you don't belong there.* Throughout my life I have fought the perpetual expectation that I have to change who I am in order to be accepted in physical activities.

When I started hiking with friends in my mid-thirties, I was predictably much slower than many. A storm of insults would swirl in my brain anytime I couldn't "keep up," and I would suddenly remember that hiking is for thin, able-bodied people with money for all the right gear. These self-inflicted insults are a result of years of conditioning by a fatphobic society that insists being fat is my own fault and I should be doing more to keep up.

It wasn't until I was in my late thirties that I was able to see past the garbage I'd absorbed from society about who is able to hike or recreate outdoors to find other marginalized folks doing activities I never thought were for people like me. Fat runners, dancers, scuba divers, hikers, cyclists, and yoga instructors were out there, and it was a glorious realization that I was not alone.

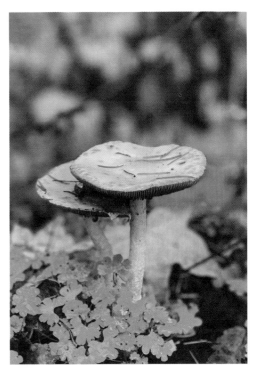

Slowness affords you time to really look at what's around you

People who are fat (or disabled, BIPOC, poor, queer, non-binary, transgender) can participate in the same activities as anybody, despite the mainstream media's usual portraits. The way in which marginalized people participate may look different from what we see in the mainstream, or it may look very similar. Some fat folks want to and are capable of running marathons, some not so much. Some fat hikers summit mountains, some not. The truth is, there is no singular way for people to enjoy the outdoors or physical activity. When I was able to allow myself to participate in physical activity in a way that met the needs of my body on any given day, my perception completely shifted. I realized physical activities didn't have to be hard or challenging or uncomfortable, although sometimes they were. I could honor the needs of my body on a hike, go as slow as I wanted, and take as many breaks as I needed. Despite what some narratives might try to tell us, there is no "right" way to be a hiker.

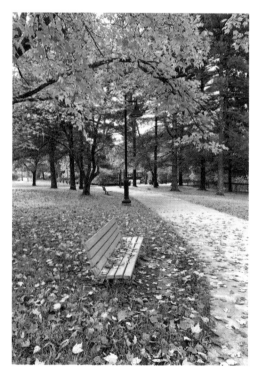

Accessible trail with a bench in Ohiopyle State Park, Pennsylvania

Joyful movement honors the body and the mind. We all have different needs. Joyful movement focuses on our inner wisdom about our body's needs and desires. We can practice honoring our bodies every day by participating in activities that nourish our sense of joy. Instead of saying, *I can't hike because I need to stop and sit every half-mile,* we can turn the thought around. First, we can acknowledge that there's nothing wrong with our need. Second, we can find accessible hikes that have benches. Third, we can purchase a portable camp stool to carry in our packs and sit whenever we need to. Fourth, we can join communities that support and celebrate our

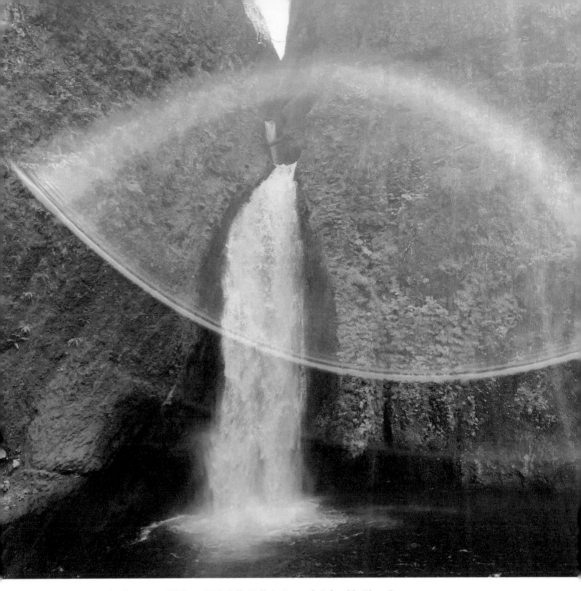

The magic of water and light at Wahclella Falls in Oregon's Columbia River Gorge

needs. Asking for our needs to be met when participating in group activities can be scary—especially if we have experienced fitness trauma—but that is why groups like FGH exist.

If we can tap into our individual needs and challenges, we find that place where joyful movement flourishes and physical activities meet the needs of our bodies, regardless of their size or ability.

BISA MILES

(she/her)

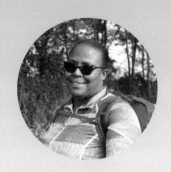

I was not outdoorsy as a kid. I am African American and grew up on the south side of Chicago on the ancestral land of the Kaskaskia, Kickapoo, Peoria, Potawatomi, and Myaamia people. Being outdoors meant playing sports, but I was considered too big and slow. So for a long time I enjoyed being outdoors in other ways—even just sitting on my front porch staring at the sky or walking outside in my neighborhood or downtown during a lunch break.

I didn't go hiking for the first time until I was forty-four years old and had finished treatment for breast cancer. I suffered from PTSD after the treatment, and being outdoors helped (still helps) calm my anxieties. I love to be around a lot of trees; it makes me feel like I'm getting a hug from Mother Nature. Once a month, I hike in the forest preserves around Chicago or plan hikes in different states or countries. In addition to my hiking, writing and travel are my big passions in life.

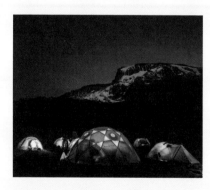

Camping in front of Mount Kilimanjaro

Sometimes people are compelled to encourage me by saying *good job*, or *good for you*—in a way that makes it clear they think I must be hiking to lose weight and make myself "better." In addition, I'm almost always the only Black person in the forest. When I do see a group of Black people, they are usually with a personal trainer. I see representation in the mainstream outdoor industry changing for me as a fat person but not as a fat Black person. That's why community means so much to me.

I hiked with the Curvy Kili Crew on Mount Kilimanjaro and with Fat Girls Hiking closer to home and found zero judgment from the other hikers. I'd hiked with another group that was supposed to be inclusive, but I didn't feel like I belonged. Instead, I felt I had to keep a certain pace to keep up.

If you try hiking with a group and don't like it, don't give up. You can find groups that have members similar to you so you won't stick out and will feel supported. I also enjoy hiking by myself—then there's no one to keep up with. If you want to try hiking alone, go on short hikes, especially to start.

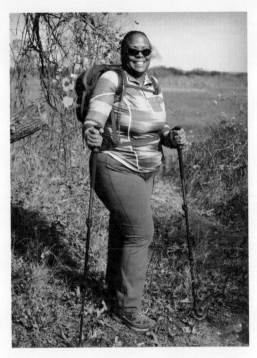

Bisa hiked Mount Kilimanjaro with the Curvy Kili Crew

When I started training for Mount Kilimanjaro, I walked around the public park wearing my hiking boots on paved concrete. The first few days of the real hike, being surrounded by trees and walking through small streams and lakes in the rainforest, brought me so much joy. It was by far the most challenging experience I'd had hiking, because I'd never hiked for five days in a row before. All my training couldn't fully prepare me for the long days, but the landscape of Mount Kilimanjaro was so beautiful, and sleeping outside under the stars so high up on the mountain was unreal—it was totally worth it.

MIKALINA KIRKPATRICK

(she/them)

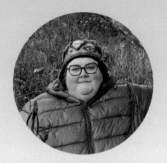

Disability-justice activist Mia Mingus talks a lot about access intimacy, the kind of intimacy you can only feel as a disabled person—or, I would argue, as anyone with a marginalized or stigmatized body—when you are with people who understand, respect, and actively, lovingly accommodate your access needs without making you feel like a burden or a token or something to pity, pathologize, or exotify. It's a place where your access needs are felt and considered to be natural, reasonable, and part of the fabric of the experience. When I think of the ideal outdoor community, I think of being with people who understand what access intimacy means; of a place where I feel safe to be open about my access needs and know that I will be heard and seen and loved and cared for; of a dynamic in which we are all really aware of each other's access needs and come together in a way that allows the person with the most needs to set the pace or the tone of the gathering; and of a place in which this accommodation is offered with love and joy and a desire to understand in an empathetic way without any shame or othering.

I love places in nature where multiple bodies of water meet and shift. Where rivers become bays and bays become the ocean. Where creeks gather to become wetlands and ponds. I love humble, low-lying places like wetlands where filtering and sifting and decomposing and renewal happens. As my body has changed over the years and I've come to live with varying levels of mobility and chronic pain, accessible natural areas that can be reached without climbing a mountain and are flat or paved and can be experienced from a chair, or even, at times, from a car, have become very important to me.

Between the ages of four and ten my family lived on thirteen acres outside of Ithaca, New York, on the ancestral land of the Susquehannock, Haudenosaunee, and Cayuga people. I was free to explore and had lots of special places where I got to know the different plants and ecosystems. Each spot brought out different feelings in me. I loved finding secret hidey-holes where I could have my own little imaginary worlds. There was a place by our driveway where a bunch of low, thick pine branches made a small cave—I'd sit inside and make potions out of twigs and seeds and leaves in an old wooden salad bowl. In the tall grass that grew in a meadow by some paper birches, I'd make tunnels and pretend to be a bunny. I explored, turned over rocks, and pretended I was living in other times and places but was also very present in the world around me. I got to know all the local wildflowers and where and when they bloomed. When I got a little older, I had my own firepit where I made fires and roasted hot dogs on sticks whittled with my pocketknife. I felt a part of nature and that nature was a part of me—there was no feeling of separation between myself and the natural world.

Just before I started fifth grade, everything changed. We moved to Asheville, North Carolina, and lived in town. We did have a backyard—it was a steep hillside with a lot of trees—but it wasn't the same. I became a town kid and started focusing my attention on other kids, as one does in adolescence.

It wasn't until I was about twenty-five that I returned to the woods and the outdoors that had nourished me in my youth. I started hiking regularly with a dear friend, several times a week for over a year. It helped me come back to myself in a big way when I was in the early stages of healing from what I now call the trauma of being born into a family with multiple generations of unhealed trauma. When our friendship changed and we didn't hike together anymore, my access to the outdoors was really limited because I didn't have a car or a driver's license and couldn't get out of town. When I met my partner, who also didn't have a driver's license, we figured out how to go camping using public transportation. For a few years, we'd pack all our camping gear (and we weren't light packers) onto buses that went close to campgrounds. I finally got my

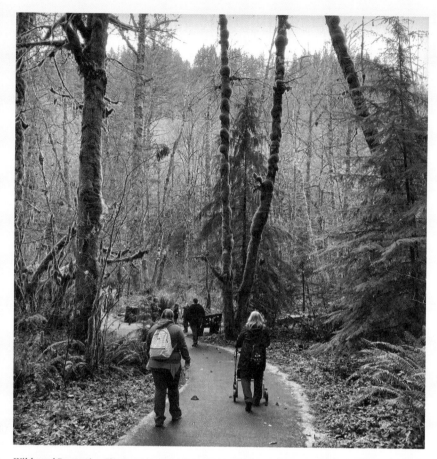

Wildwood Recreation Site

driver's license in my mid-thirties, and access to nature was one of my primary motivations.

My physical disabilities impact my ability to walk without unbearable pain. Sometimes I can, sometimes I can't, but we always find ways to be outdoors. I have a very sturdy folding stool with a high weight capacity that can fit in a regular backpack in case I need to sit down and there are no benches. I have a wooden walking stick. I have large comfy folding chairs for times when I just want to sit and watch the trees and the birds. These days, I don't do what I call *hiking*. In my mind, *hiking* connotes going up a hill or mountain or walking a particular distance. Most people similarly define it as how high and how far, and that way of thinking doesn't work for me. I've had to let go of it and it's been really freeing.

I go outdoors to reconnect with myself and with nature. To reconnect my head to my body, to process and integrate, to move my body and feel myself as an alive being, and to let go of the conditioned fear and alienated relationship I've had with my body, which still needs to be healed and reclaimed regularly, as a practice. I go outdoors to remember who I am and who this being we call planet Earth is, and to feel my physical self and mental aspects as part of the larger body of life and universal being.

At times in my life, it has been very hard for me to be outdoors, and I did not enjoy it. Before I started healing my relationship with my fat and later disabled body, I experienced a long stretch of time in which being outdoors felt like something I was failing at. I've had times in my life when my body seized up in such a way that I couldn't walk without experiencing excruciating pain and numbness. For a while, one of my legs "forgot how to leg," as I put it—I couldn't hike, couldn't climb the mountain, couldn't even walk down the street without suffering. It felt like another sign that my body was a failure—that I'd failed at having a body.

At other times, I have found it very hard to be alone with myself and my thoughts. Being outdoors and in nature can put you in direct contact with your inner world, and if you're not ready for it, if you're hurting and feeling shame and anxiety and don't know how to sit with those feelings with gentle self-compassion, getting outdoors and exploring your connection to creation can be overwhelming.

I can go for long periods, months sometimes, when I'm really struggling or busy or in a lot of pain or a deep depression, and I don't remember what being outside feels like beyond going between doorways and my vehicle. At other times I might be walking in nearby parks or sitting in my backyard almost every day—or driving out to the coast, to the mountains, or to the pond once a week. It ebbs and flows. Allowing myself to have this variation is an important part of my healing, both from the circumstances of my individual life experience and from living in a traumatized and traumatizing culture. I find that as I continue to heal, I'm able to be more aware of what being outdoors does for me, the medicine that it is, how much I need it, and how to prioritize it into the rhythms of my life, whatever those rhythms may be at the moment.

There aren't as many accessible outdoor spaces as there could be— specifically places with flat, paved trails with seating at regular intervals or close to the parking lot. I'm always so grateful to find trails that are accessible to people who use mobility aids like chairs, scooters, walkers, and canes, or paths that are accessible to people who can't climb mountains or need a place to stop and rest from time to time. It's especially difficult to find these accessible trails in areas outside of towns and cities—we long for places that have an immersive feeling of wildness to them, where we can feel close to the untamed parts of ourselves. Equally challenging is finding places to swim or be in water that don't require a scramble up and

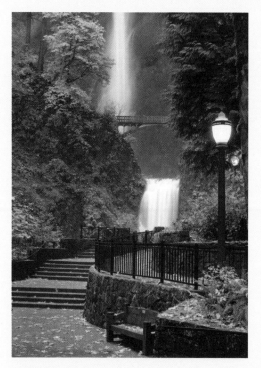

Multnomah Falls near Portland, Oregon

down a steep riverbank. Because finding these places that meet my combination of needs can be challenging, I usually do a lot of online research and ask for advice from people with whom I share access intimacy.

So much about outdoor activity is framed in a really performance-oriented way. For many years as a fat person, an aging person, and a person experiencing chronic pain and growing disability, I found it difficult to overcome my own internalized shame enough so that I could reach out to other people with whom I could spend time outdoors.

I think it's so important to mention self-acceptance, acceptance of personal limitations, and how our abilities and bodies change over the course of a lifetime. As my body changed over time, my abilities changed—accepting that, and learning to adapt in order to create accessibility for myself, was a crucial step that allowed me to reclaim my personal access to the outdoors. So much of my realization of this dream had to do with releasing body shame and healing from traumas that alienated me from myself—I needed to understand the landscape of accessibility and self-reclamation on a personal, political, and even spiritual level.

Finding a fat-positive community, disabled community, and body liberation community was another key component of the journey. I needed people who got it; people open, comfortable, or thoughtful enough to consider my accessibility needs without making me feel patronized or pitied (I have a really sharply tuned radar for that). While some of the barriers I've faced have been about the internalization of external stuff, I do experience bigotry from people outside these communities.

First, let me acknowledge that when people come across me outdoors, they see a white person. I've never experienced racial bigotry. People may or may not perceive me as queer. So I experience a lot of protection from the very real dangers many others experience due to bigotry, hate, and ignorance. Still, people have a lot of opinions and prejudices about superfat and disabled folks. These opinions and prejudices are communicated in subtle, often subconscious, and unexamined ways. It could be a look of surprise or even disgust on a trail, a full once-over with someone's eyes, or double or triple takes. Though these acts are silent, they are a form of communication, and it's a message I receive loud and clear.

Then there are people who say things like *way to go* or *keep going* and offer unsolicited feedback that I know they wouldn't offer someone who wasn't fat. These comments are based on preconceived notions absorbed from a fat-phobic culture about what it means to be in my body and why I might be moving it. They assume I'm trying to lose weight. The people who talk to me like this have all kinds of ways of communicating this expectation and tell me not only what they think about it but also how they are qualified to "help" me.

Sometimes these things get to me and sometimes they don't. The deeper I go into my own self-acceptance, the less often it affects me, but I do have vulnerable days. Sometimes, on days when I'm feeling the most vulnerable, when I could really benefit from being out in nature, I choose not to go out into the world because I don't want to deal with other people's bullshit. This happens in all movement spaces. I love the water, and I love going to the pool at my community center, but I have experienced some of the worst health trolling and people showing their preconceived notions about what it means to be in my body from supposed well-meaning people in the pool and locker room.

If you want to know how welcoming the outdoor community is, you'll need to be specific, because the answer very much depends on whom you're asking, where you're looking to be welcomed, and what your access needs are. There are gatekeepers who do not greet every body gladly. There are people who do not want to be associated with or make space for every body. There are people who work at agencies who decide what kinds of trails are going to be built, whether or not there are accessible features, and whether or not that's important. In some places it's clear that accessibility matters to the people who designed the human interfaces. In other places not so much.

A competitive, performance-based culture exists in the outdoor world as much as on the football field, it just has a different flavor. I will not feel welcomed by that mountain. But if I go to the path that gently rises and falls along the river that collects snowmelt from the same mountain, it's a whole different story. The metaphor of the mountaintop is a big one in our culture. Don't get me wrong, I love the experience of being in a beautiful place and getting to experience sweeping views from a high vista. But the mountaintop metaphor is burdened with connotations of conquering, domination, struggle for struggle's sake, planting a flag, and being the best or the first. It's one of the ways mountains get climbed in our culture. Fortunately, it's not the only way.

There are so many other exhilarating and meaningful perspectives we can take in, absorb, and learn from. I think it's crucial for white people especially to seek out those experiences where we aren't attempting to

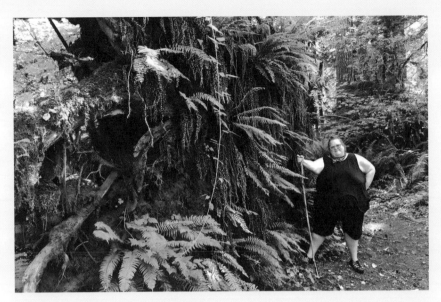

Mikalina hikes with a wooden stick for stability

get to the top of the mountain but instead paying attention to what it means to be interconnected with other beings—to be a part of something rather than on top of something.

When I look back at the story of my life, my love of being in nature started very young. As a toddler I loved being naked and outside, and I loved finding summer mud puddles to "swim" in. I was totally enchanted with flowers and bugs and worms and water and stones and everything alive. My love of nature is something I've returned to and reclaimed over and over.

If I haven't been outdoors in a while, a sticky clogged up feeling overtakes me. This internal reminder inspires me to reconnect with the beauty of the life and death cycles that are so apparent and visceral outdoors—even if all I have the capacity for is to sit outside and smell the decaying leaves, feel the wind on my face, and hear the sounds of neighborhood scrub jays and crows from my backyard. Being outdoors is always, in the words of Mary Oliver, "announcing your place in the family of things." That inspires me. That reminder. To hear that announcement over and over.

WILDWOOD RECREATION SITE
WELCHES, OREGON

Mikalina Kirkpatrick (she/them)
FGH chapter: Portland, Oregon

The Wildwood Recreation Site along the Salmon River in Oregon has paved accessible paths and oodles of benches to rest and reset my body when I am in pain. My favorite spot is the cattail marsh—you walk down a long boardwalk built over the wetlands and into an open marsh to stand (or sit, there's a bench there) suspended above this amazing environment. It feels incredibly immersive. In spring, the redwing blackbirds have nests among the cattails and you can watch them feed their babies tiny green worms and listen to them calling to each other. Small snakes bask in the sun on the boardwalk in summer and woolly bear caterpillars do the same in fall. There are little purple-leaved aquatic plants floating on the surface of the marsh year round. Cattails were a big part of my childhood, and being among them reminds me of my early relationship with nature. It's wonderful to get this reminder of my childhood home, which is all the way on the other side of the continent.

DISTANCE ROUND TRIP Cascade Streamwatch Trail is a 0.75-mile loop. The Wetlands Trail is a 0.75-mile loop.

ELEVATION GAIN Cascade Streamwatch Trail gains 39 feet. On the Wetlands Trail, the trail grade is less than 8 percent—hardly any elevation gain at all.

CELL SERVICE Spotty and unreliable

ADA AND GENERAL ACCESSIBILITY The trails and facilities at Wildwood Recreation Site are ADA accessible. Benches are spaced close together on the Cascade Streamwatch Trail.

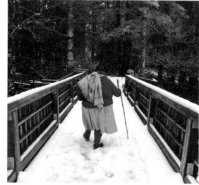

Mikalina visits this area often, in all seasons

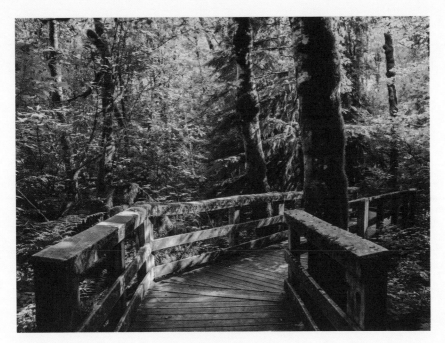

Boardwalks throughout Wildwood Recreation Site make for a fun, accessible hike

BATHROOMS Yes. There are ADA-accessible, all-gender bathrooms at the trailhead and other parking lots.

NATIVE LANDS Confederated Tribes of Grand Ronde

TRAIL DESCRIPTION The Wildwood Recreation Site is thirty-nine miles east of Portland and surrounded by the Mount Hood National Forest. It is open year round and has over five miles of paved, accessible trails, picnic areas, and lots of benches. There are recreation facilities, wetland ecosystems, forested areas, accessible interpretive trails, and boardwalks, and some parts of the trail parallel the Salmon River. The Cascade Streamwatch Trail features an underwater look at the Salmon River, fish habitat, and river conditions, while the Wetland Trail features a cattail marsh with an opportunity to view birds and other wildlife.

OFFICIAL PARK ADDRESS Wildwood Recreation Site, E Highway 26, Welches, OR 97067

TRAIL NAME The Cascade Streamwatch Trail and Wetland Trail

HOW TO FIND THE TRAILHEAD The trailheads have signs and are easy to find from the parking lots. There is a $5 fee to park.

BUGS AND HUMIDITY

OR WHY I DIDN'T START HIKING SOONER

Bugs and humidity—ew.

Growing up in rural Minnesota, I decided early on that it wasn't much fun to be outdoors except within a cumulative time-frame of about four weeks in spring or fall, otherwise known as the Midwest sweet spot, in which it's warm and there's no humidity and no bugs.

Picture the scene: It's a winter day in northern Minnesota. Kid-me and several of my cousins and siblings announce to the adults, *We are walking to the island!* Our Grandma Ruby has a house on the shores of Island Lake, named for the small island at its center. Kid-me has never been on the island. It is mysterious and cool, with trees and no people, and we really want to walk on the frozen lake without adult supervision. It seems like a glamorous adventure.

Better bundle up! one of the aunts hollers. We put on too-big snow-mobile suits, winter jackets, snow pants, hats, mittens, and boots then penguin-walk out of there, down Grandma's long driveway, to the boat launch and onto the frozen lake. A white wonderland stretches out before us. We follow some truck-tire paths through the deep snow. There are several ice houses for fishing in the distance. We're slow and one cousin cries—it's hard to tell who since we're all so bundled up. Someone pees their snow pants and we barely make it past where the docks would be in summertime. At least we tried.

Yes, we get a lot of snow in Minnesota. But that's not the most challenging part. It's the cold that sucks most. Do you know what wind chill

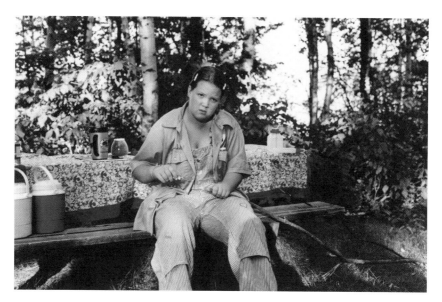

Me at sixteen on a family camping trip in 1995

is? If not, you likely grew up in a moderate to mild climate without such worries as your nose hairs freezing together or the fun game where you throw a glass of water in the air and it comes back down as not liquid. It's a terrifying kind of cold, and, needless to say, not a climate I really wanted to tromp around in. I mean, there are many fun things about snow—tubing, sledding, snow forts, snow people, the quiet magic of it all. I miss the snow in my everyday winter life. But I appreciate it more now that I have to drive a few hours to the mountains to see it.

Summers in Minnesota aren't much better. Imagine you're a kid in the 80s and you think, *hey, I'll put on my swimsuit and lay out in the sun—put some baby oil on my skin, spray some Sun In on my hair, and stretch out on the dock at grandma's lake with a magazine.* Sounds fun right? Wrong. This is a summer fantasy and the humidity laughs at you for being sucker enough to even try it. Regardless of anything you do, you're sweating profusely. Your body is sticky. There is no escape. Sitting in the shade, motionless, there's sweat on parts of you you didn't even know could sweat, like behind your knees. I hate sweating. I hate when I walk and it feels like swimming through soup. I don't know a more eloquent way to describe it. Hot soup. Ew.

And finally, I have saved the best part of the Great Minnesota Outdoors for last—mosquitos. The joke in Minnesota is that the mosquito is our state bird. It's truly no joke though how many mosquitoes there are in that lake-logged state I love so much. Mosquitoes will annoy you at any time of the day, but dusk always seems to be the worst. Swarms of the tiny bloodsuckers can surround you and make you wish you'd stayed inside (luckily, I've recently developed a new and better sense for when they've landed on me, and though I know they're essential to their ecosystems, I've gotten really good at slapping them dead). We were always told using a fingernail to make an X on the bite would keep it from itching, but it's not the most successful relief, especially if you're covered with bites.

When people ask me why I only recently began to enjoy the outdoors, I refer them to the aforementioned points. It took me a while to realize that not every outdoor environment is plagued by some variation of these personal deal breakers.

We didn't have a lot of money when I was growing up. We were poor. There were five kids and one mom in our family. We all did our share to take care of one another, cook, and clean (although my older sister insists that she "raised me" and she's the second mom of the family—she's only two years older than me!). I wanted to make my mom's life easier. She worked hard, often at two jobs, and also went to school. My siblings often tease me, saying I used to ask mom, *Can I clean the house again?* I admired how hard she worked. It couldn't have been easy with all of us, but she did an amazing job of ensuring we had what we needed. We relied on food stamps and the food shelf often. We went to garage sales and thrift stores for our clothing and household needs or got hand-me-downs from friends and family. It didn't occur to me that these things weren't common until kids at my school made fun of my secondhand clothes and glasses from the welfare box at the eye doctor.

While my dad paid child support from the comforts of his big fancy home, we'd be guessing the contents of label-less dented cans from the food shelf. When my sister and I went to visit our dad in the city, it was a wildly different experience from life at home. I felt so disconnected from life at my dad's house. I wasn't allowed to be myself there. He would ridicule the way I looked—from my hair and glasses to my clothes. There was always something I just couldn't get right.

Dad worked as an agent and scout in the modeling industry. It was literally his job to criticize and judge the way women and teen girls looked. He was good at his job and very successful in his field. My sister and I would often hang out at his office in Chicago, pouring over Cindy Crawford's look book and coveting the life of Niki Taylor or Tyra Banks. My chubby weirdo self never measured up.

City life interested me because of the people, culture, and tall buildings, but the places that fascinated me were faraway lands without humidity or mosquitos or brutal winters. Mom took us on vacations we could afford. Road trips to visit one of our aunts in Montana were some of my favorite times with my family. We got to witness new landscapes, see horses up close, and learn about ranch life. Once, we went on a road trip to Grand Canyon National Park. I remember standing before the vast never-ending majesty of the canyon at one of the scenic viewpoints and thinking, *It snows in Arizona?* I mean, I also thought it was beautiful, incredible, and awe inspiring, but sixteen-year-old-me had so little real-life travel experience that there was a lot I had yet to learn. I felt small and insignificant, but with a sense that the world had a lot to offer. The idea of all that possibility seemed scary at the time.

One summer, we took a family camping trip to a lake somewhere in northern Minnesota. It was a small lake with no motorized boats and an anchored platform with a ladder to get out of the water off shore. Though I had brought a stack of books to read (I still do this when camping), I mostly swam. I liked to swim underwater. The submersion and quiet appealed to me. The water in that lake seemed pure and clean. When I was underwater, there was no hum of faraway boat motors, just a slight tick and the breath I exhaled around me. I learned to dive off that platform, practicing over and over. I know I slept in a tent, but I don't remember if it

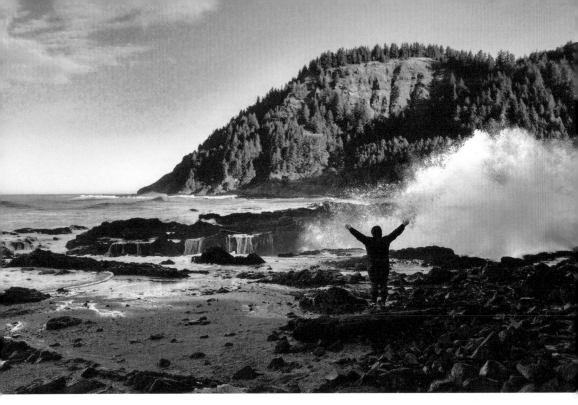

Cape Perpetua on the Oregon coast

was with my siblings or my mom or if I had my own tent. I don't remember what we ate or what was cooked for meals or if we had a cooler even. I just remember the feeling of the water around my body and the quiet nights among the trees.

When I moved to Oregon in 2008, I was reluctant to go on hikes. *Everyone* seemed to be into hiking and the outdoors here. In spite of some of my lackluster beginnings with nature, I begrudgingly went on a few hikes near Portland. It took several years of these sporadic outings before I finally realized that hiking was something I could actually do. Bonus, Oregon wasn't particularly buggy, cold, or humid. Hooray! Once my love of hiking in Oregon solidified, I felt confident exploring other places and trails. Now, when I go home to Minnesota to visit my family, I research hikes. I have found some great gems I didn't know existed when I lived there. It's pretty magical to be able to introduce your self-declared non-outdoorsy family to beautiful nearby places in nature.

SUMMER BROWN

(she/her)

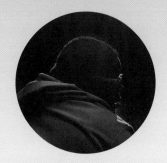

Growing up, I didn't really know a lot of people who did outdoorsy stuff. I loved splashing in puddles and digging in the dirt, but I didn't really like getting dirty. I have been fat since I was about seven, so I often shied away from physical challenges. I went to a summer camp in high school, but I didn't go camping or hiking until I was a teenager. When I moved to Washington State in 2010, I started camping more regularly. My ideal place to be outdoors is somewhere warm, but Pacific Northwest weather doesn't always allow for it. Since I hate being cold, anyplace around a firepit sounds good to me.

More than everything, I've always enjoyed just being near water. I love sea creatures and wanted to be a marine biologist when I was a kid—until a trip to Sea World where a dolphin bit me! Still, I love the water and the beach. I feel grounded when I'm outside, especially when I'm near water. I love the colors and the sounds of nature. I love trees. I love adventure and exploring new places and having new experiences. Even though it's cold here in winter, summer in the Pacific Northwest is gorgeous—I love when I can chill in my hammock in the backyard.

I'm used to taking up space where I'm unwelcome—I'm fat, Black, and queer—but I do wish the outdoor industry would upend systems of oppression that entitle certain bodies over others. An inclusive outdoors means everything from eye contact on trails to more accessible hikes and campsites to simply making space for people who have different needs and look different from those the mainstream outdoor industry has led us to expect outside.

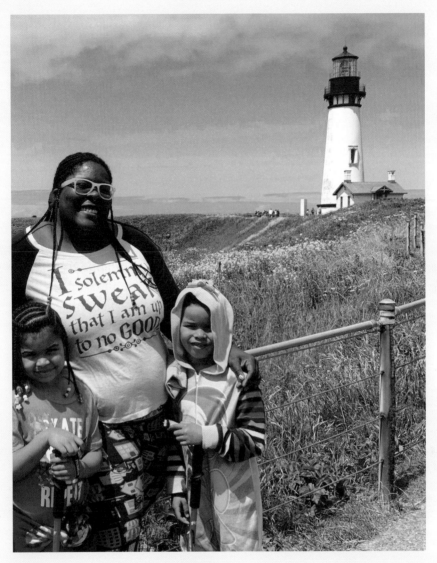

Summer on the Oregon coast with her twin kiddos

Today, I am a marriage and family therapist and a writer who is passionate about supporting the wellness and healing of marginalized people: BIPOC, queer and trans folks, disabled folks, fat folks. My kids inspire me to get outdoors (even if it's cold out). Their joy and wonder around the natural world creates a space of healing and happiness for me.

GRAND TETON NATIONAL PARK
WYOMING

Summer Michaud–Skog (she/her)
FGH founder

Grand Teton National Park has some of the most incredibly scenic mountains, lakes, and wildlife. There are countless places to pull off the road into parking areas where you can take in the landscape—it is one of the most breathtaking places accessible by car. But if you want to get out of your vehicle onto a trail, there are several ADA-accessible options in the park. Jenny Lake was most impressive to me because it has a wheelchair-accessible trail that goes right up to the lake and lots of benches. Plus, the views are stunning, the lake is clear, and there are rangers available to answer any questions or curiosities you may have about the area.

DISTANCE ROUND TRIP The ADA-accessible Jenny Lake Trail is half a mile, with the option to add on additional trails that are not ADA accessible.

ELEVATION GAIN Elevation on the ADA-accessible portion of the trail is minimal.

CELL SERVICE No cell service. The seasonal visitor center has WiFi.

ADA AND GENERAL ACCESSIBILITY A wide, paved trail from the parking lot parallels the shore of Jenny Lake, with many benches along the way.

BATHROOMS Yes. There is an all-gender, ADA-accessible single-stall toilet near the parking lot.

NATIVE LANDS Cheyenne, Eastern Shoshone, and Shoshone-Bannock

TRAIL DESCRIPTION The Jenny Lake Visitor Center, campground, and other facilities are open May to September. The ADA-accessible trail along Jenny Lake is paved, with many benches for resting and a spot along the lake that allows for wheelchairs to be rolled right up to the water's edge. The majestic mountains and clear lake can be seen from the trail as you meander through the forest. Beyond this accessible section of the trail, there are more trails to the visitor center, around the entire lake, and beyond.

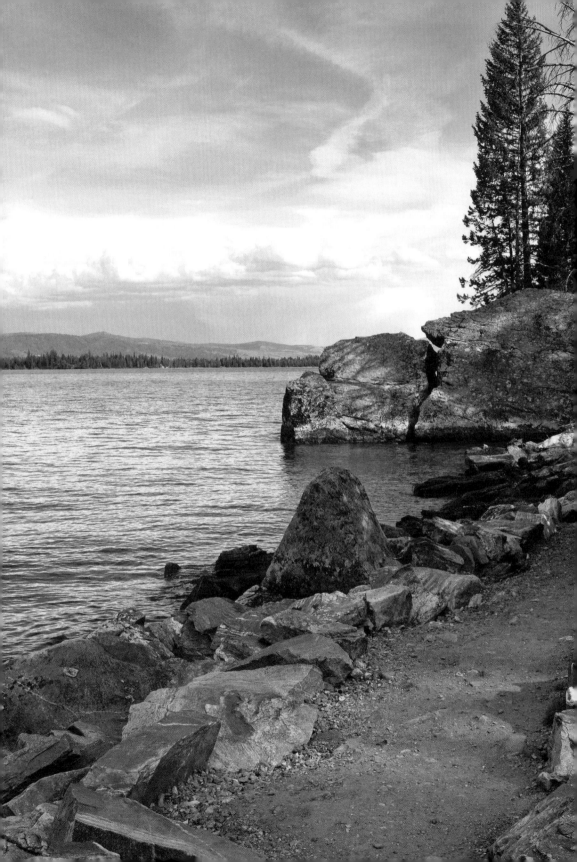

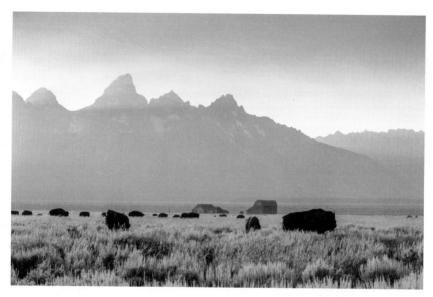

A bison herd in Grand Teton National Park, Wyoming

OFFICIAL PARK ADDRESS Jenny Lake Visitor Center, Teton Park Road, Moose, WY 83012

TRAIL NAME Jenny Lake Trail

HOW TO FIND THE TRAILHEAD Park in the Jenny Lake parking lot and follow signs to the trailhead. At the trailhead there are maps of the area that indicate the ADA section of the trail.

SUMMER'S HIKING TIPS There is an ADA–accessible boat shuttle near the trailhead that (for an additional cost) takes you across Jenny Lake to the base of Teewinot Mountain and to more trails (although the trails on the other side of the lake are not ADA accessible).

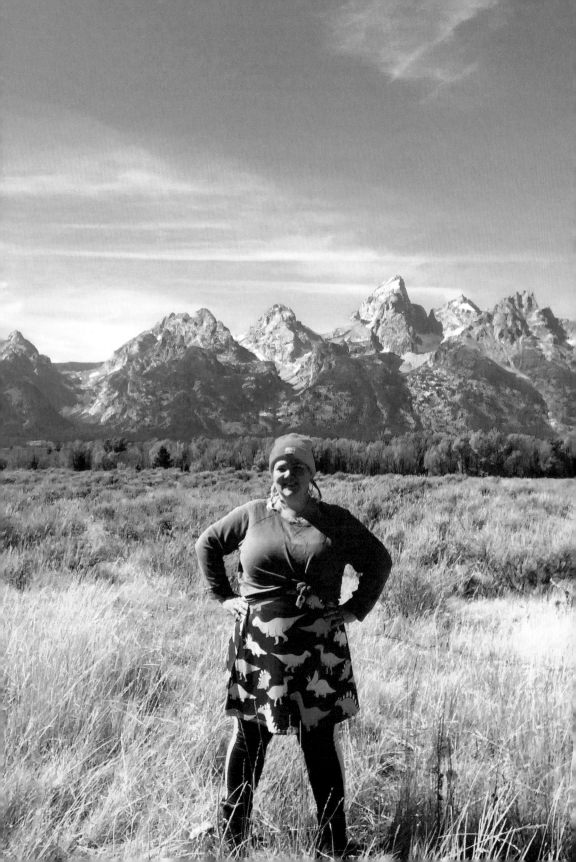

AMANDA G

(she/her)

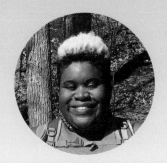

At seven years old, I went on a camping trip with a well-known organization for girls to learn outdoor skills—instead I learned that I wasn't welcome in the outdoors. There were only three Black girls in the group. All the other girls slept in brand new tents. Us Black girls were given a crappy tent that was basically a tarp with a flap. It rained that night, and we got soaked. Even at that young age, I knew why we ended up with that tent—I knew we didn't belong in the outdoors. This racist experience led me to write off camping and any organized outdoor activities for a very long time. Mostly, I would stick to playing outside in rural southwest Virginia with my cousins on bikes and four-wheelers. In summer, we were beach people.

In third grade, my school was near a wooded area, and at recess, my teacher encouraged me to cross the baseball field and go down the hill to check out a gravel wooded trail through the forest. The Wood Trail opened onto a field full of weeds and had lots of places to explore and get off the path. It was a great place to be outdoors. When I decided to get back into hiking as an adult, I wanted to re-create the experience I'd had on the Wood Trail as a kid.

When I went to college over two decades ago, I sought to be part of the outdoor culture there, but it felt exclusive. The college I attended was classist, racist, and homophobic, and it was a challenging five years of my life. The college has often been a source of trauma and inaccessibility for me, but recently, I returned to the area and went on several hikes. I even climbed to the top of a nearby mountain. After the hike, I was reminded of good times I'd spent watching meteor showers on a hill behind the campus golf course. I found myself healing by returning to a place that held a lot of my trauma and discovered a lot of joy being back there.

In the work I do now, I support and advocate for first-year college students and underrepresented students. My aim is to radically redefine and change the academic system for these students through advocacy so I can offer them a better experience than what I had in college. I help students with marginalized identities explore their passions and strengths. I also help them navigate the "hidden curriculum"—those lessons that aren't listed on the syllabus, but that every student absorbs anyway, including values, norms, perspectives, and attitudes. This advocacy and the work I do toward creating systemic change in the university structure to support equity and justice in education is my life's passion.

My other passion is weightlifting. I started with CrossFit in 2013 but got injured in 2015. A year later, I reconnected with fitness, focusing exclusively on weightlifting and joining a local gym with a Black coach.

Weightlifting is divided by weight class, and I started competing as a super heavyweight. At a competition, another heavyweight competitor approached me and introduced herself as "the other super heavyweight" competitor. This interaction inspired me to create a community of big strong athletes. I made fliers for a community of super heavyweight lifters called Big Girl Barbell, a fat positive fitness space and community, and handed them out at my next weightlifting competition. I also created the Big Girl Barbell Instagram account, where I repost videos of people competing or practicing. Big Girl Barbell is not only a place for fat people to see themselves represented in athletics, it's also a place where we can talk

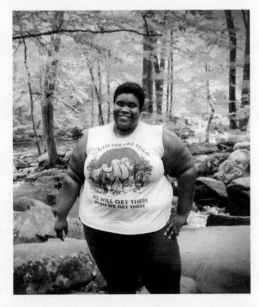

Amanda gets there when she gets there

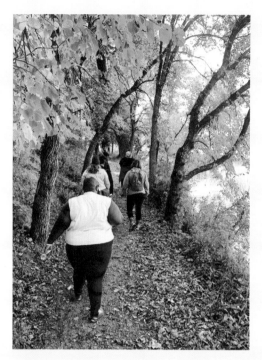

Amanda on a group hike in Minnesota

about race, racism, fatphobia, and sexism in athletics. I love that we're changing the narrative that there's only one type of person who can be an athlete or an outdoorsy person.

When I get outdoors now, I often want to challenge myself to do something difficult. I like to know that I can do it. I want to find new obstacles and move my body through spaces to understand how it moves. I love how hikes challenge me and remind me of my strong sense of self-reliance and creative problem-solving ability. I lean into body trust and feel empowered. I typically spend time outdoors every three weeks because I have found that I physically and emotionally need that time to recover. The time in between, I sit outside by my firepit and enjoy the nature around my home. I also lift weights at my gym. Typically, it's gym during the week and hiking on weekends.

I do a lot of research and preparation to avoid bigotry in the outdoors. If I find a hike that I like online, I will research it on YouTube to see who is there and what the terrain and people look like. Is it socially safe? I always find the location on a map. Will it be safe for me as a fat Black woman to be in the woods there? You never know who is going to be out on the trail. I lose some of that wonder and discovery of a new place with these preparations, but this is how I feel comfortable in the outdoors. And when I feel comfortable, I can push off internalized fatphobia and find people that look like me hiking too.

I try to anticipate the challenges and fears that might come up in any new activity or experience. When I name my fear, stand in the fear, address the fear, and face the fear, I am able to ask myself what I can do to get past the fear without minimizing it. Is the fear based on past experiences? I honor that and then I ask myself what I need to make happen so I can have this new experience. I research, prepare, and make a plan for self-protection and safety.

I've found that hiking with supportive and encouraging people has made my experiences in the outdoors better—luckily, the internet has allowed me to connect with like-minded hiking buddies. The outdoor industry's focus on colonial mindsets like "conquer mountains" and "discover the wilderness" is not welcoming. Popular outdoor gear stores don't help fat people, because they don't have gear to fit us. That exclusivity creates a toxic culture. But the outdoor industry and mainstream outdoor culture is irrelevant to me when I can find pockets of community for fat folks and Black folks online.

When I get outside, I'm reminded that, regardless of what the "industry" does, Black people have always been outdoors. There is so much forgotten and untold history. Thankfully, conversations around equity and diversity are happening. People who are typically cut out of the conversation are creating new spaces—not only connecting in real life and on social media in meaningful and amazing ways but also challenging individuals and corporations to do better. In the meantime, my husband and my dog give me all the support and space I need to move in the ways I need to move and rest when I need to rest. And I have found the confidence to hike on my own.

The freedom I feel, deep in the woods with trees and birds—I don't feel that in everyday life. There might be just five minutes when I feel completely free and safe, but those five minutes are worth being hot, or deflecting the stigma of heavy breaths or the people who might think I don't belong. In those moments, I'm transformed back into a content and carefree third grader hiking through the woods during recess.

KOHLER-ANDRAE STATE PARK
SHEBOYGAN, WISCONSIN

Shayna (they/them) and Callie (she/her)
FGH chapter: Milwaukee, Wisconsin

SHAYNA: As a kid, forests were a fantastical place of wonder for me. I would imagine the elves and fairies that could be out there, just out of sight. As my adult life got busier, I made less time to get outside and started to lose my connection to nature. It wasn't until I moved back to Sheboygan and reconnected with the great Lake Michigan (and went on my first FGH hike) that I remembered everything I'd been missing—the crisp Wisconsin air, the sounds of cawing birds and crashing waves, and the sense of oneness with everything and everyone around me.

CALLIE: I found my love of hiking while at a retreat in Vermont in 2008. I still remember my first ever on-top-of-the-world feeling after finally making it to Buttermilk Falls. That was the start of my break-up with diet culture and learning to practice gratitude for all that my body does for me (even though some days are more of a struggle than others).

SHAYNA: As someone who has lived in the Sheboygan area for most of my life, I can't believe it took me so long to find and fully appreciate this hidden gem of a trail. I was always drawn to the forest paths in the park, preferring the overhang of trees and the smell of damp soil in fall. But after trying my hand (and feet!) at the dunes, I was hooked. Sometimes the trails are a little sandy, making for slow going, especially while going downhill on some of the steeper dunes. Sometimes the uphill climbs—which look relatively short—leave me begging for a pause. I'm always rewarded with a stunning view of the lake, which I like to soak in while sitting on a bench. The sounds in the dunes are a unique blend of rushing air, cawing seagulls, and the rasp of waves along the shore. I always loved the orchestra of the forest, but there's a unique comfort in breathing in time with Lake Michigan's crashing waters.

Each time, the trail looks just a little bit different—from small shifts, like new plants cropping up—but mostly, there's a timeless quality to it all. Lake Michigan is always there, waiting to listen to whatever you may want to say. The gulls never stop

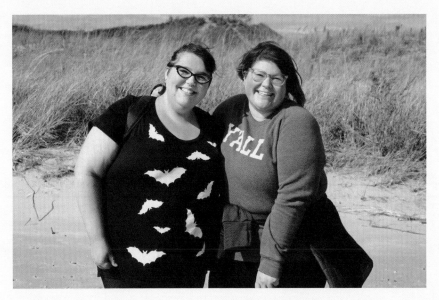

Shayna and Callie lead FGH group hikes in the Milwaukee, Wisconsin, area

calling, soaring up into the sky, and diving down toward the water. The shrubs and trees that nestle in the sand shimmy and sway. There's a peace to it all that can be hard to find in the city.

DISTANCE ROUND TRIP About 3 miles, depending on the route you take

ELEVATION GAIN 88 feet

CELL SERVICE Spotty and unreliable

ADA AND GENERAL ACCESSIBILITY This trail is not ADA compliant. Because it's built on sand dunes, there is often sand on the trail, especially on windy days, and in small sections the wooden boardwalk is totally obscured by sand. Since there are generally no rails to hold onto, take your time and go slow where you need to. We strongly recommend wearing shoes with grip. There are a number of benches for resting along the way.

BATHROOMS Yes. In the Sanderling Nature Center (when open) there are gendered bathrooms that are not ADA accessible.

NATIVE LANDS Menominee, Myaamia, Potawatomi, and Sioux

TRAIL DESCRIPTION The Dunes Cordwalk Trail will take you over the dunes along Lake Michigan, where you can watch the waves roll in, the seagulls over the water, and the

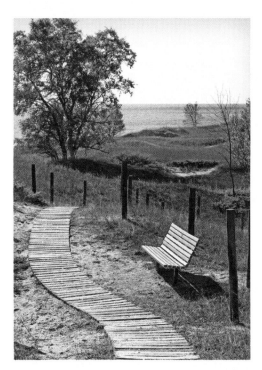

Benches along the boardwalk are great for soaking in the sights and sounds of the dunes

lively forests nearby. Expect an often-sandy wooden path with much-appreciated benches dotted along the way, especially at the tops of the dunes where you can overlook the water. You'll have the option of circling back either along the trail itself or on the beach (as long as the water levels aren't too high). If you're able, we highly recommend walking back along the beach to get your toes (or fingers) in the sand and admire the washed up driftwood and plethora of stones that have been smoothed and rounded by the waves.

If you're tired and want an easier walk back, there's also the option to return along a road. When you reach the end of the path, you'll find yourself going through a small area of trees before hitting the paved Old Park Road. Be sure to watch for cars here! If you turn right and walk a short way, you can turn right again on Beach Park Lane, which will take you back to the nature center parking lot. There are bike lanes on either side, so you can walk on the grass next to those (if you walk on the bike paths, keep an eye out for bikers trying to pass). Cars typically give pedestrians and bikes a wide berth, but make sure to stay alert if walking back this way. You'll pass a lot of beautiful foliage on this route and can expect a smooth walk back.

Despite this being a rather popular trail, it never feels busy. You might pass by a few families, but most of the time you'll feel like you're the only one on the trail. After your hike, we also recommend stopping in at the Sanderling Nature Center if it's open. They have recommended ideas and interactive displays to help you learn about the area, not to mention a cool gift shop.

OFFICIAL PARK ADDRESS Kohler-Andrae State Park, 1020 Beach Park Lane, Sheboygan, WI 53081

TRAIL NAME Dunes Cordwalk Trail

HOW TO FIND THE TRAILHEAD Kohler–Andrae State Park is about two miles south of Sheboygan on County Highway V. You can find it easily on Google Maps but cell service is unreliable, so be sure to look up directions before you start driving.

Once in the park, you'll round a corner to where you can either pay for the day, buy an annual park sticker, or continue on if you already have one. Typically, it will indicate that you pull ahead past the booth and park to go inside to make your purchase, but watch for the signs indicating if you should do this or stop at the window. From there, continue driving forward until the first left turn, Sanderling Lane, which will bring you to the Sanderling Nature Center parking lot. While the trail can be started from a point farther down, we recommend starting here.

SHAYNA AND CALLIE'S HIKING TIPS This trail is great for kids. Not only will you see other families along the way you'll also find a lot of fun learning opportunities, especially if you stop in at the Sanderling Nature Center first.

Check the lake's water levels before you start so you'll know ahead of time if you can expect to take the beach back or not. Unfortunately, the water is high more often these days than ever before, so the beach may not be available during certain times of year.

BODY LIBERATION AND NATURE

_

THE POWER OF WORDS

have been called fat for most of my life. The first time I can remember was in elementary school. Three girls always picked on me for how I looked and what clothes I wore. One weekend, I got a perm at my grandma's house (it was the 80s—kids got perms), and I was excited to go back to school with my new look. In gym class the first day back, we played volleyball or dodge ball or some game with a ball, and one of the girls said to another, *Ha! Look at Summer! She looks like Shirley Temple.* The other girl responded, *No, she's too fat to be Shirley Temple, she looks like Medusa.* They called me Medusa for years after that. It stung. I was so ashamed.

From a very young age, girls are told, both implicitly and explicitly, that the way we look is something people can use to harm, discredit, and shame us. Society bases our value, worth, and personal security on how attractive or pleasant we look to others. It places value on our bodies according to how they conform to arbitrary aesthetics and functionality.

Diet culture is a system of beliefs that values thinness as an ideal body type and encourages weight loss, disordered eating, and exercise to achieve the idolized body type by any means. It affects every facet of our society and is upheld by all the systems of oppression woven into that fabric, including white supremacy, patriarchy, colonial standards of beauty, capitalism, gender norms, and cisheteronormativity. Diet culture is steeped in ableism, racism, classism, sexism, and shame, and it equates thinness to a person's moral virtue.

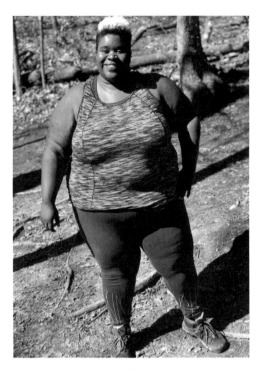

Amanda, founder of Big Girl Barbell, finds joy in both hiking and weightlifting

Fatphobia is defined as the fear of fat, fat people, or becoming fat. It is a cog in the wheel of diet culture, as is anti-fatness. People of all sizes are affected by fatphobia, but people in fat bodies are the ones who face oppression, stigma, bias, and discrimination. What I experienced in gym class was fatphobia and anti-fatness, but I didn't know that at the time—all I felt was deep shame for who I was. Anti-fatness shows up in interpersonal relationships, online, in school, at work places in every single industry, at home, and in medical offices. Internalized stigma occurs when fat people absorb the anti-fat ideas they hear and see and begin to speak to themselves in the same ways that the wider culture does.

When diet culture is firing on all cylinders, we learn from very early on, as children if not as babies, how high (or low) our social and cultural currency is. This value is based on biological and genetic traits—things that are, for the most part, completely out of our control. If the standard is to be thin and our body doesn't fit into that standard, we will be reminded repeatedly, through media, advertisements, television shows, movies, and anywhere else humans are represented, that we aren't worthy of respect.

Historically and still today, fat people are the punch line. Those joke tellers (and anyone who shames another person for being fat) often believe that fat people *choose* to be fat through overeating and inactivity. These same people believe that if fat people wanted to badly enough— if we just worked hard enough and had some discipline—we could lose weight and become socially acceptable and also, "healthier."

But the truth is, fat people can't be shamed into being thin. Fat people don't owe anyone proof that they are healthy in order to be respected. And some fat people will never be "healthy" based on cultural standards. Health is defined as being free from disease or illness. For folks with chronic illness or disease, the cultural definition of health is not attainable. In addition, the shaming, oppression, and marginalization of fat people causes much mental, emotional, and spiritual distress, yet these mental health factors are rarely considered when we talk about what it means to be healthy. For a long time, I believed those who told me that my mental health wasn't as important as doing whatever I could to be smaller.

I have tried a few times to be less fat through diet and exercise. Each time I lost weight, I gained it quickly back. What's more, any time I intentionally changed the foods I ate or the type and frequency of the movement my body did, my joy was lost. I like food, and I am active, but when I would spend time worrying about calories in or out and force myself to go to the gym, I was miserable. I never felt better when I lost weight. Never. I felt empty, shallow, vapid, and hungry. The weight loss was never, ever, sustainable. The change in food or movement was never, ever, sustainable.

These days, I would rather cherish and honor my body as it is. I'm just naturally fat, what's the big deal? People are naturally thin and society never calls those bodies an "epidemic."

The word *fat* makes some people uncomfortable. People often want me to use an easier word. Plus-size. Curvy. Chubby. Big. Fluffy. These euphemisms are fine for some, but I don't use them. I say, *I am fat,* because that feels the most true to me.

Please, just let me use the word. I self-identify as fat. It's no different than identifying as a woman or queer or white. Despite cultural stigma, the fat identifier is inherently neutral. In addition to the cringe response from strangers, there can be a lot of emotional labor that goes into conversations about identifying as fat. Fat liberation and anti-diet culture are not subjects everyone knows about. I constantly gauge whether or not people are open or ready to really listen and whether or not I may get anti-fat feedback or uninformed comments. When I share a photo online of myself on top of a mountain or at the river, unapologetic in a bikini, with my big, round, soft belly uncovered, I'm aware that it may get negative reactions. I post these photos that some consider "unflattering" as a way to unlearn the bias still alive within me and as a fuck you to diet culture.

Fat is a descriptive word for someone's body type, but it's also a radical reclamation of bodies deemed unruly by our beauty and body-obsessed culture. The real stigma isn't the word itself, it's the way our culture puts blame on people for having the nerve to be fat—as diet culture has taught us, our bodies are out of control—fatness can and should be contained with determination, diet, and exercise. If only we had more willpower.

When I say, *yeah, I'm fat*, it really upsets folks who would rather have fat people stay silent in their shame and try everything in their power to become thin(ner). Happy fat people are a threat to those who blame their own body for their unhappiness, insecurity, and dissatisfaction with their lives. How many times have you heard someone in your life (maybe you yourself) say something like, *If I could just lose x amount of weight, I would finally be happy*? This idea is everywhere. As with many types of oppression, there is a system that benefits—an entire industry makes billions of dollars off body shame and the cultural hierarchy of bodies. The implication is that we cannot claim happiness until we have attained a bodily ideal (set by our own standards or society's, usually whichever is smaller). So, how dare I use the word *fat* in a positive way?

I like the subversive, radical, rebellious nature of using the word *fat*. I find reclaiming a word that has been used to harm me empowering, and I'm proud of rejecting the stigma and shame associated with it. But empowerment isn't enough.

Any time I wear my FAT BABE t-shirt, I am keenly aware of where I am and who is around. I've had people shout things like *Fat Fuck!* from their cars at me when I wear that shirt. Sometimes I just don't have the energy to justify my own existence and my right to describe myself as I see fit.

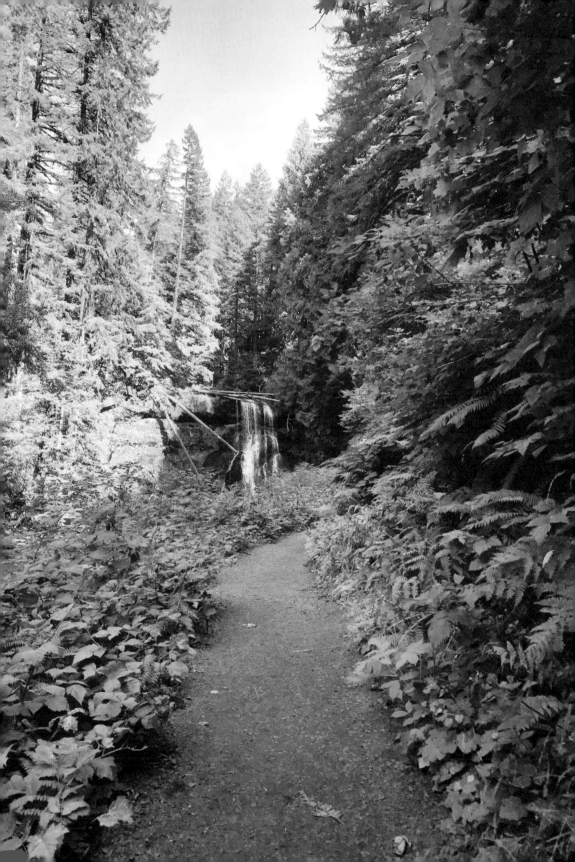

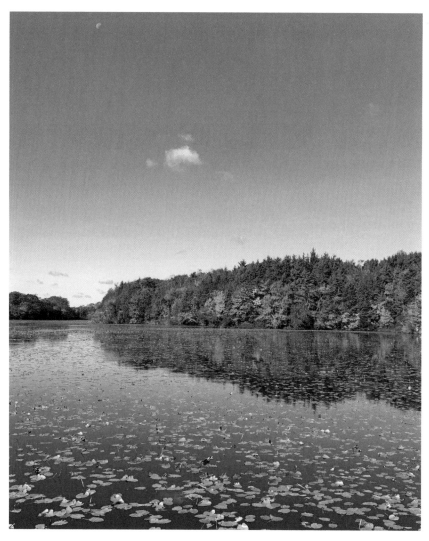

Fall in New Jersey

My formative years were difficult at times, but they gave me strength. I forged a path to body adoration that, without a doubt, lead down trails lined with old-growth trees and waterfalls, deep in the forests of the Pacific Northwest. I didn't know my body's strength and resilience until I put myself in situations where I had to rely on my intuition, knowledge, and creative problem solving to get my fat body from the trailhead, through the woods, and to the destination.

I learned to trust my body. I learned to trust myself. I spun myself around, head thrown back to look up at the canopy of trees overhead, and much of the shame society placed on my body fell away.

I'm fat and I want to be considered a "real" hiker. When I first began hiking on a regular basis, it seemed like a label I wasn't allowed to claim. Hikers look a certain way, I was told. Hikers have certain gear, I was told. Hikers traverse a specific landscape, distance, and elevation gain. Even though I went on hikes that challenged me and continued to hike farther than I'd ever gone before, I couldn't be a real hiker because I was fat.

Research and knowledge were integral to building my confidence and making me comfortable enough to call myself a hiker. In the beginning, I would see numbers on hike descriptions and not understand what they meant. When I read that a popular Portland hike was "1600 feet of elevation gain in 2.5 miles," I didn't know what that meant in terms of how steep the hike was or how long it would feel for my fat body with chronic pain. All I knew was that I would do my best, listen to my body, and honor my needs.

I would often be sweaty, out of breath, tired, and the slowest person on the trail, but when I made it to the summit or waterfall or whatever my destination was, it always felt like another seed of trust planted within me. The hike back down felt like growth. I would be so happy, I could hear romantic-comedy-happy-ending music in my mind. I was goofy, silly, chatty, and giddy. Those endorphins carried over into my everyday life. My body confidence grew as my hiking confidence grew. I began to crave the outdoors and made a places-to-hike list. No matter where I was, I yearned for the long paths along forest creeks the color of evergreen trees. It no longer mattered to me what I looked like or what gear I had. Or what people said about me. The only mirrors in the outdoors are the ones that self-reflect.

As my own confidence and radical rejection of diet culture began, those still under its spell tried to pile shame at my doorstep again. Some acts of oppression are small, micro-aggressions that don't feel right, like the *good for you* comments only directed at the fat people on the trail. Other comments are more overtly oppressive, like the health-concern trolls who want to share future health outcomes for my fat body. If only I would lose weight, then I wouldn't be such a strain on the health-care industry. As if the healthcare industry has ever given a shit about fat people.

Our culture pushes fat people to the margins. A lack of representation, plus-size clothing and gear, and accommodating physical spaces (chairs, bathroom stalls) are all forms of marginalization. Discrimination and weight-based stigma deny fat people access to many aspects of society.

Systemic oppression is easy to ignore and deny if it doesn't affect you personally, which is why community is so important to cultivating understanding, validation, and healing. The concept of "body positivity" began as a radical movement. It was created by fat, Black women. But thin, white women co-opted the term, turning it into a diet-entrenched space that marginalizes the very people who created it.

I no longer use the term *body positive* to describe the work I do. It's clear to me that the work I do with Fat Girls Hiking is fat activism. Fat activists are still figuring out the best language to describe our work. *Fat positivity* centers the fat body, but some activists have moved away from using the term *positivity*, as it creates an unrealistic ideal that we must always feel positive about our fat bodies. *Fat acceptance* is a term used by activists to create a broader, more neutral understanding for folks living in bigger bodies.

In my own activism, I gravitate toward the terms *body liberation* and *fat liberation*. Body liberation recognizes the need for distance from diet culture's toxicity and freedom from the societal, cultural, and systemic oppression anyone in a marginalized body faces. Fat liberation recognizes the specific intersection of folks in fat marginalized bodies.

Bodies everywhere exist on a spectrum of sizes, and that's no different in our fat communities. I am a midsize fat woman, which means I can usually find clothes in stores and mostly (sometimes painfully) fit in seats

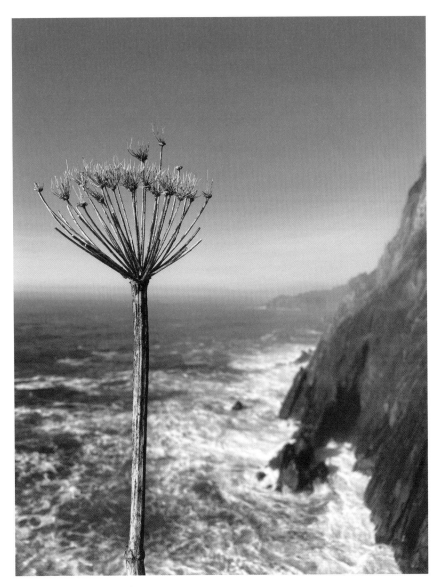

An ocean-view hike never disappoints

and physical spaces. I have been fat shamed on trails, faced weight-based bias in medical settings, and endured endless micro-aggressions in real life. However, I don't face the same severe and blatant daily bullying as

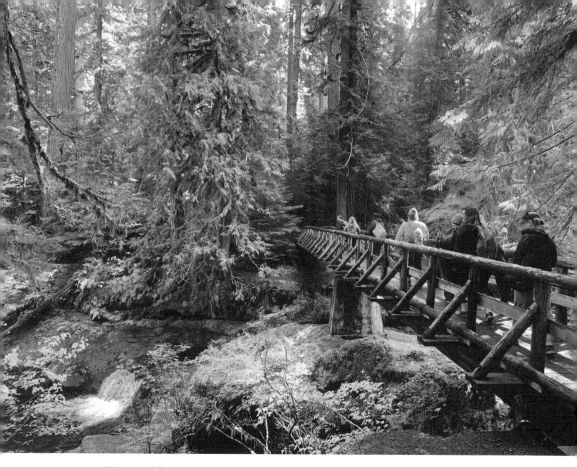

FGH group hike, Mount Hood National Forest, Oregon

folks in bodies larger than mine. The spectrum of fatness is important to note because the experience of someone who wears a size XL will be vastly different than of someone who wears a size 7X. Access to clothes, public spaces, and basic needs become even more of a challenge for fat folks at the bigger end of the size spectrum. Ash, creator of *The Fat Lip*, has pioneered important work on the fat spectrum, and I defer to her podcast on the subject.

When I am outside connecting with nature, I'm able to heal from the oppression I face daily. The stress, anxiety, and challenge of living in a world that feels like it's not made for me fade when I watch ocean waves predictably arch and curl and break on the shore. My body belongs next to a mossy 100-year-old cedar tree that overlooks a creek where salmon swim upstream every fall. I exhale the burden of shame in heavy breaths as I walk uphill. Every wildflower, fungi, and leaf is a gift. I can take all the time I need to contemplate their beauty. My body fits perfectly here, on the muddy path lined with fern, hemlock, Sitka spruce, and Douglas fir so big and old they make my body feel small. When I am next to the ocean, a mountain, a waterfall, I can see how insignificant I am, size-wise, in the grand scheme. A sigh of relief comes over me as I marvel at the beauty of the bigness we celebrate in the natural world.

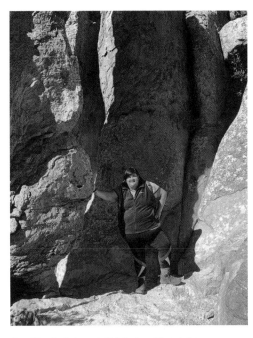

Amy Rios in Arizona's Chiricahua Mountains

A place in my mind knows that the vastness we crave from vistas, oceans, mountains, and the outdoors in general is really a need to remember our connection to and see ourselves reflected in the natural world. The old-growth trees standing strong and resilient remind me that my thighs are my trunks and I can sway with the breeze. The long fissures and dimples on the beach caused by waves and wind remind me that the stretch-marked skin on my fat body is part of nature. The view from the mountaintop goes on for miles and reminds me of my bright inner world, full of dreams.

My goal is to help every fat person find peace in the knowledge that there is room enough in the outdoors to celebrate however our bodies show up. We can carry that knowledge with us back to the trailhead, to our cars, to our homes, to our communities, to our culture and tell them all, *We deserve to be here!* Our fat bodies are reflected in nature, and when we behold our inner worlds and open the door to healing, we are liberated.

MINNEHAHA FALLS REGIONAL PARK
MINNEAPOLIS, MINNESOTA

Summer Michaud–Skog (she/her)
FGH founder

I often visited Minnehaha Falls as a kid, teenager, and adult when I lived in Minnesota. I would climb down to get a better view of the falls and marvel at them when they froze in winter. Waterfalls have always felt soothing to me. It wasn't until 2017, when I led a hike for the FGH community, that I got to experience the trails around the falls. The limestone rocks in the area are marvelous and the fall foliage is incredible. I love that the hike ends where the creek you've been hiking along joins the mighty Mississippi River. It's a hike right in Minneapolis so there's easy access to the trail system. Unfortunately, you can expect to find a certain amount of trash, graffiti, other people, and noise, but, regardless, there are moments of calm and peacefulness to be had here.

DISTANCE ROUND TRIP 1.8 miles

ELEVATION GAIN 167 feet

CELL SERVICE Yes

ADA AND GENERAL ACCESSIBILITY The trail is not ADA accessible—there are stairs—but a wheelchair-accessible viewing area is available above falls, and it has benches.

BATHROOMS Yes. ADA-accessible bathrooms are available in the park nearby.

NATIVE LANDS Wahpekute and Sioux

TRAIL DESCRIPTION This well-known and much-visited waterfall is right in the heart of the Minnehaha neighborhood of south Minneapolis. Paved paths take you from the street to the viewing platform of

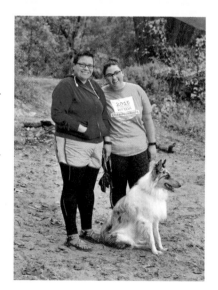

We love dog-friendly trails

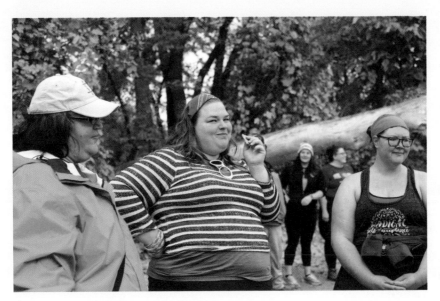

A group hike from Minnehaha Falls to the Mississippi River

Minnehaha Falls, a 53-foot waterfall that cascades from a limestone cliff. Take the stairs down to view the waterfall before starting down the Minnehaha Creek trail. There are dirt trails on either side of the creek with periodic bridges that connect them—take one trail to the Mississippi River and the other on the way back to create a fun loop hike. The trail parallels the creek through forest to the confluence of the Mississippi River where there is a sandy beach.

OFFICIAL PARK ADDRESS 4801 S Minnehaha Drive, Minneapolis, MN 55417

TRAIL NAME Minnehaha Creek Trail

HOW TO FIND THE TRAILHEAD You can find Minnehaha Falls Park on any digital map or GPS. Park on the street, in one of the pay lots, or arrive via the nearby bus or LTR lines. Walk through the park and follow the signs to the waterfall where you'll also find the trailhead.

SUMMER'S HIKING TIP Bring a trash bag on your hike and leave the trail better than you found it. Rent a bike or grab a snack at Sea Salt Eatery in the park.

MARLEY BLONSKY

(she/her)

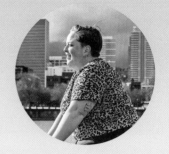

I grew up in the suburbs of Fort Worth, Texas, on the ancestral lands of the Kickapoo, Jumanos, Tawakoni, Wichita, and Comanche people and spent most of my free time playing outside. I rode bikes with the neighborhood kids until sundown, climbed trees into a little fort we built, and made mud pies with locust skeletons. I was also fortunate to attend a camp nearly every summer from first through tenth grade, so I was well-versed in good environmental ethics and stewardship from a young age. Many of my favorite memories are camping with my mom or dad—we'd paint rocks, wade in creeks, and roast s'mores. But I hated to exert myself and dreaded hiking, long walks, or strenuous activity. I loved to learn new skills at camp, like archery and canoeing, but never wanted to be competitive at them. These early interactions made a lasting impression on me and affected my relationship with outdoor activities as an adult. I'm still hesitant to go on super-strenuous adventures, because I like to do things that I know I'll be successful at and within my body's capabilities.

In 2014, I got really into biking and bike camping. I was twenty-eight, freshly divorced, and searching desperately for a way to connect to my body and emotions again. I started commuting to and from work by bike, found a community that rode together socially, and was introduced to bike camping and bike adventures. From there, it's been a whirlwind—finding a bike that I love and that fits me, finding clothing that fits properly (a huge challenge), and making a place for myself in the bike world. My passion in life is riding bikes and connecting with people. I feel fortunate that my work as an environmental manager helps fund my passion and provides time and opportunity to travel.

A few years ago, I was invited on a three-day group bikepacking trip with a Portland-based women's cycling team. I knew I was going to be the only fat person on the trip, but checked out the route and felt confident about it. The ride ended up being much more challenging than I was prepared for, physically and mentally. I was hungry for a lot of it, cold and wet, and doubting my abilities to keep up with the group. After an honest conversation, we realized that a few of us were struggling and were able to reset the group expectation. From then on, we had a much better experience. I was still physically tired—it was by far the most challenging physical ride of my life—but mentally, I felt supported by the group.

Adventure is the main reason I get myself outdoors—to see things and to clear my head. I'm a restless person so being outside lets me appreciate everything there is to see. I also struggle with depression and anxiety, but on my bike, I feel like I can think clearly and get the demons out of the way. On my bike, I am able to meditate, connect to my emotions, listen to what they tell me, and respond appropriately.

There have been times in my life when my ability to go outdoors has been limited by external factors (wildfires, illness, weather), and I notice an immediate impact on my mental health. Even if it's as simple as working from an outdoor location or eating dinner outside, I need the fresh air to rejuvenate my soul. I have a corporate eight-to-five job, which keeps me tethered to a computer most of the time, but I've made it a priority to take breaks outside, even when the weather is not so good. I've found that even a quick walk around the block, or a bike commute on the rainiest of days, is enough to keep my spirit going.

As a noncompetitive, fat cyclist, who rides for fun and adventure, I have never seen myself represented in mainstream outdoor media. People always assume that because I'm fat, I must be a beginner. I want to be 100 percent clear with this statement—there is absolutely nothing wrong with being a beginner, and a lot of my advocacy work is about bringing new people into cycling. But the automatic assumption at bike shops or on group rides that fat people are novices or beginners, just because

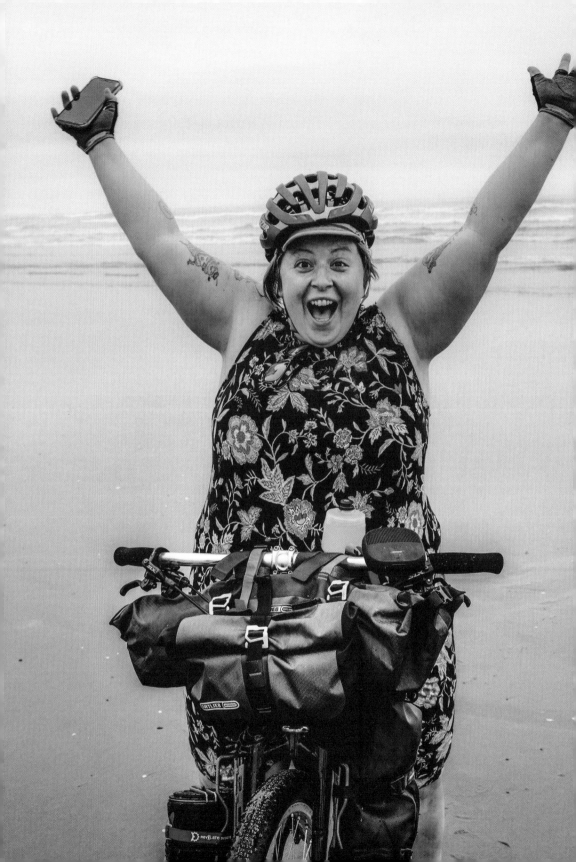

of our body size, is insulting. Because fat people don't fit the image of outdoorsy people as svelte and tan, when people encounter us outdoors, they're surprised and don't know how to react.

The biggest barrier for me as a fat cyclist is finding appropriate clothing and gear. Sure, for many of my rides, especially shorter and more casual rides, I can wear nontechnical, everyday clothing. But many of the rides I enjoy are longer and would be greatly improved by bike-specific performance apparel (such as a bike jersey and bottoms with a chamois). Wearing an ill-fitting kit can lead to chafing, saddle sores, and other discomforts, as well as constant adjusting on the bike, all of which sucks. Also. I'm not waterproof. But I've yet to find a cycling rain jacket for fat people. This is immensely frustrating.

Things are getting better, representation-wise, for fat and marginalized folks in the hiking community and general outdoors industry, but the bike world remains elusive. I'm confident that change is coming though, especially with the current Covid bike boom. The bike industry is waking up to the massive untapped market that is fat folks, and I think we'll start to see improvement soon.

Biking and bike camping and adventures are possible for people in bigger bodies. You have absolutely nothing to prove to anybody. If you want to ride, go ride. Your life is yours to live, and yours alone.

VERONICA MIRANDA

(she/her)

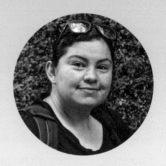

I volunteer with Latino Outdoors as their program coordinator in the San Francisco Bay Area. I'm passionate about connecting people to the outdoors and sharing beautiful spaces through photography. The mountains are my medicine. I love walking under a canopy of trees and seeing the sun shine through the forest. It's beautiful and eerie at the same time. When I'm outside, I'm filled with curiosity and a sense of exploration—it improves my mental health. I love visiting open spaces to observe the ecology, learn about an area's Indigenous people, and photograph the

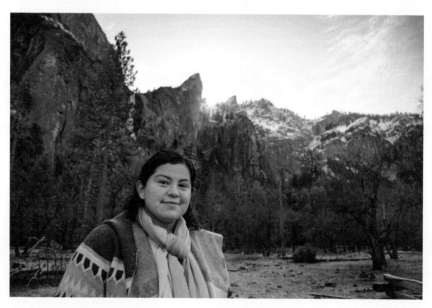

Veronica in Yosemite National Park

beauty I see. Getting outdoors helps my brain detox from all the chaos that is going on at the moment.

Access and knowledge are the biggest barriers for people getting outdoors. Some parks can't be reached via public transportation, which is an issue for people who don't drive or can't access a car. Not all parks are ADA friendly, and it can be difficult to find information about which are and which aren't. In conversation, I've noticed certain recurring barriers that keep people in the Latinx community from enjoying the outdoors. Some have simply never heard of the open spaces nearby or don't know how to access them. Others aren't sure what they'll need to bring to enjoy a day hike or how to read a map. Not knowing where to go or what to bring makes people feel unsafe. I believe everybody deserves a community that gives them the confidence to explore outdoor spaces for recreation and mental health.

I wasn't much of an outdoorsy kid. My family would visit the beach or lake every now and then, but my childhood consisted of mostly local parks and playgrounds. In fourth or fifth grade, I went to science camp. We took a school bus up to the Santa Cruz mountains in California. It was the first time I ever sat around a campfire or saw a banana slug—it was pretty fun. Whether playing on a blacktop during recess or in a local park, I have always loved the fresh air while outdoors.

When I met my husband (almost fifteen years ago!), he helped me start hiking. He's an avid outdoorsman and enjoys camping, fishing, and hiking. When he would bring me to his favorite outdoor places, their natural beauty just blew me away. I was instantly hooked.

I am a slow hiker, so I take my time. I used to stumble a lot, but I've since found my footing, and now I'm more confident. Hiking at high elevation is so challenging—it still gets to me. Not everybody outdoors is welcoming. I've had people give me dirty looks on hikes—I think because of my size and the space I take up. On a narrow trail, I can be harder to pass, which bothers some people. I remind myself that we all deserve to enjoy the outdoors, no matter how much space we take up.

My husband (and now our kiddo) inspires me to spend time in nature at least three to four times a month. We go to the beach and hike or go car

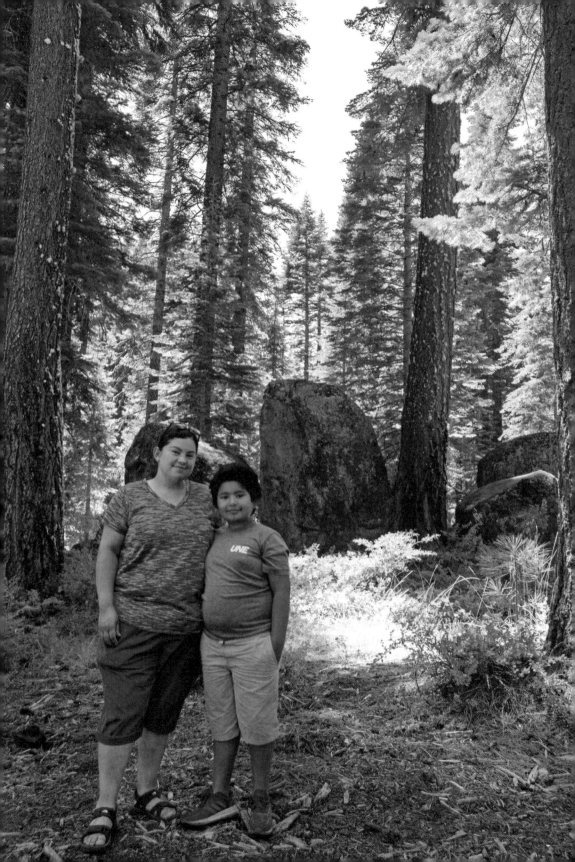

camping. Watching my son become comfortable outdoors and aware of the space around him makes me ecstatic. I love that I can feel confident allowing him to run up ahead of me on a trail and be safe around a campfire or an axe.

Recently, I have seen a jump in BIPOC folks in outdoor-marketing campaigns, which is awesome, but I feel the larger-bodied community is still not represented. I don't see fat folks in ads or promotions or even on information signs or literature at parks. Just the same ol' thin, able-bodied folks. It's unfortunate because fat people go outdoors too.

The more you visit outdoor spaces, the more confident and knowledgeable you become. It may be scary at first, but the beauty you'll find is totally worth it. If you're nervous, reach out to someone you trust and ask them questions, read books or magazines about the outdoors, follow outdoorsy people on social media, or join a local outdoor group that will make you feel safe and comfortable.

TAMERA

(she/her)

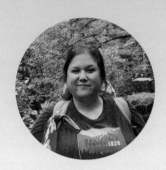

I have hiked for as long as I can remember. I was a very outdoorsy kid, who grew up on the ancestral land of the Cherokee people in eastern Tennessee and western North Carolina, and would hike, swim, and fish in the creeks. *We're going on an adventure*, was something we said a lot growing up. While outdoors, we'd try to find different wildflowers to identify, collect rocks, spot turtles, and catch tadpoles. A lot of my childhood memories surround the outdoors in some way.

Recently, I discovered that the creek behind the property of my grandparent's house in Asheville, North Carolina, flows from there into other creeks and is eventually connected to a river that flows near where I currently live in Knoxville. This connection from one place that holds so much importance to me to another that I value immensely makes me weep. I feel that connection in my heart, in my DNA, not only because it is the land of my ancestors but because of my personal history with the land. I can't fully comprehend or articulate why the Smoky Mountains are so important to me, but I do know that this deep connection to the land my family comes from helps me maintain a deeper connection to myself.

I like to hike by myself because it gives me time to listen to my own body and intuition. As a woman alone, I'm more afraid of men in the outdoors than I am of a bear or a rattlesnake. When I come across a man or a group of rowdy men, I always brace myself for harassment or unwelcome comments. I trust my intuition to keep me safe, but the prospect of hiking alone does sometimes make me worry about what I will do if I have an emergency of some sort where I need to rely on strangers who aren't friendly. I always protect myself while in the outdoors, but I wish it wasn't something I had to consider.

I've had some really great moments hiking alone, but I've also had some challenging ones. Once, after I'd completed a hike I've done many times, I returned to the trailhead and met a couple who hadn't started yet. They asked how long the hike was, and when I answered they seemed surprised. They said something like, *Oh, well good for you, that you get out and try to exercise.*

Another time I told some people about how I'd made my fastest time on a trail I've hiked many times. To which they said, *imagine how much faster you could hike if you lost weight.* My proud moment faded. Because of fatphobic comments like these, I used to worry a lot about what I looked like or how people saw me. I subscribed to their diet culture ideation and started to think about how many calories I might burn on a hike. There was no joy in hiking for me then.

I needed to ask myself some tough questions. Why was I wasting my energy? Hiking is not about burning calories or losing weight. It's about connecting with nature. It is something I love. I went to the top of that mountain, and I was fat all four times I hiked it.

Reminding myself of why I hike and all that hiking has given me quiets the negative self-talk. Whenever I struggle on a trail, I stop and look at the moss, trees, and rocks and find joy—the real reason I'm hiking.

Community helps with this too. In addition to hiking alone, I also hike with older people, and I love the pace and carefree attitude they offer. It's important to me to have people in an outdoor community that I can relate to and who understand the level of difficulty for trails in the same way I do.

Representation matters, and I enjoy seeing fat people doing different things in different places. The outdoor industry has some work to do on this front. It's important to remember the established outdoor industry has its own culture, but it isn't necessarily the only way to spend time outdoors. The industry has a long history of exclusion, and they have a lot to do to make up for their past. As a fat woman, I have never been able to find outdoor gear that works for me. My whole life, all my gear has had

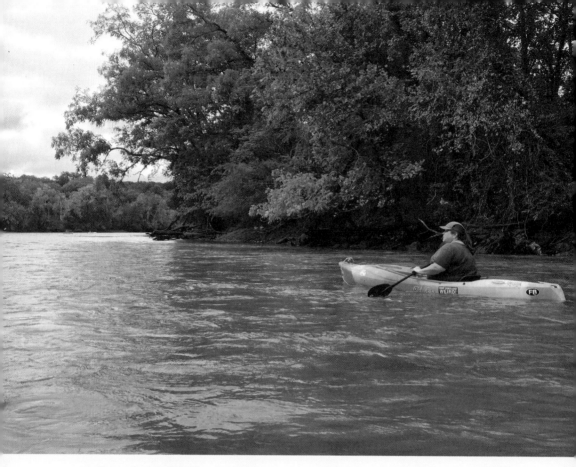

Tamera has been kayaking since 2014

to be adapted. It simply isn't made for me. At the same time, the industry invests a lot of time and resources into making you think you have to have the right "stuff" to get outdoors and hike. It's no surprise that fat women are afraid to explore outdoor recreation—the cards are stacked against us.

It can be easy to be discouraged or afraid to try new things because it's hard to be what you can't see. A fat woman in a kayak is not something I'd ever seen, but it turned out that the first time I got in a kayak I took to it like a duck to water. In 2014, some very supportive family members encouraged me to join them on a ten-mile paddle on a mostly calm river. I was so excited to try it, and a big part of that is that my family let me know what to expect. It was important and encouraging to have people who could show me what to do and be kind about it. I used my aunt's extra sit-on-top kayak, and, despite my worry that I wouldn't be able to find a life jacket that would fit, I ended up borrowing one that fit perfectly from a neighbor.

Water grounds me. I enjoy time on my kayak more than anything. I love skies, panoramic views, flowers, moss, fungus, and all the elements. I live my life with the motto *find beauty in the small things*. When I can slow down, stop, and appreciate my surroundings, it helps me remember the possibilities that are present every day if I keep my eyes open to them. When I am out on the water, it feels so natural, like I'm finally where I belong.

Learning how to set my expectations accurately has been instrumental in helping me enjoy my time outside. I like to ask myself, *What do you want to see when you're outdoors?* I don't always know the outcome of every situation, but I'm not afraid to push myself into new experiences. I give myself little goals—two or three things I may want to do or see while outdoors—but I don't feel bad if I don't accomplish them. Start small with your own goals. Keep it real, and remember—no one gets in and out of a kayak gracefully.

VAN LIFE
ON THE
MARGINS

REDEFINING SUCCESS

I was a kid in the 1980s. A time before the internet and social media. A time when photos of missing kids were on milk cartons. A kid my age from the small town next to mine went missing. Turns out, he was a friendly kid who was in the wrong place at the wrong time.

Because of things like this, my mom was a stickler for our safety. She taught us how to be independent and empowered. One of our favorite cassette tapes, *The Safety Kids*, came with a coloring book on how to make safe choices. Songs like "How to Memorize Your Phone Number" and how you should "Find a Grandma or Mother With Children" if you get lost in a grocery store, and, my favorite, "Stay Outside of My Line," a song about body autonomy and telling someone you trust if an adult touches you inappropriately. I still get these songs stuck in my head, which means they were an effective tool. Being a kid in this era also involved horror stories about "stranger danger" and predators in vans who offered candy to kids as a lure to trap them. We knew better. Mom taught us to stick together and look out for one another. We were Safety Kids.

I moved to Minneapolis when I was twenty years old. It was exciting to be around so many different kinds of people. My mom would come to visit me, and I noticed how she would chitchat with pretty much everyone. It used to really annoy me until I realized: I'm the same exact way. But my childlike inner brat wondered, *Whatever happened to stranger danger? Does that just go away as an adult?*

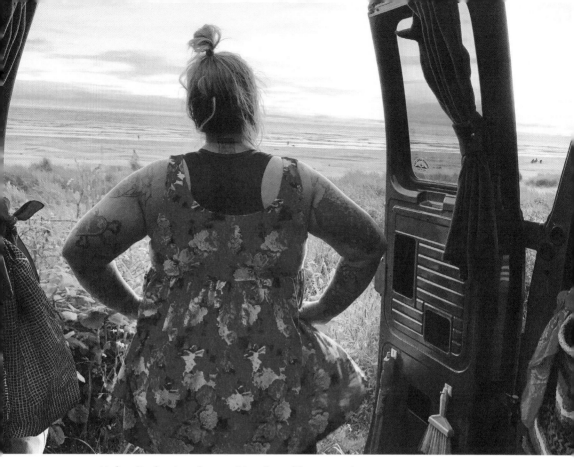

My favorite place to park my van? Anywhere with an ocean view

I eventually learned that safety is relative depending on who you are. If you're a marginalized person, your idea of safety is probably different from that of a person with privileges. I navigate the world as a white person, which grants me access and safety in many places. I also travel as a woman alone, which poses certain threats to my safety. I mostly pass as a straight person, so being queer and lesbian is something I have the privilege of divulging or not to strangers depending on how safe or unsafe I feel that decision will make me. Chances are, if you've never had to wonder if you're safe, you have multiple privileges with which you walk through the world.

As a queer woman in this world, I am constantly aware of my safety when I'm around other people. When I'm out on a trail, I think about my safety in a multi-layered way—there's bears and cougars and snakes, and there's also people. People have inherent biases and prejudices that could jeopardize my safety. I'm a fat, queer woman, alone on a trail. But my white privilege can often override the parts of my identity that are marginalizing.

In spite of sometimes feeling unsafe, you kind of have to talk to strangers when on a trail. It's awkward if you don't. Because, often, you're the only humans in sight—if you don't at least say hello, it's just weird.

People in the outdoors are typically friendly. I have had overwhelmingly good experiences on trails from people I pass or stop to chat with. I love this aspect of hiking. I meet people I normally would never come in contact with. However, I have also encountered anti-fatness and sexism and feared holding my girlfriend's hand on a trail. Yes, the outdoors are for everyone, but not everyone experiences them in the same ways.

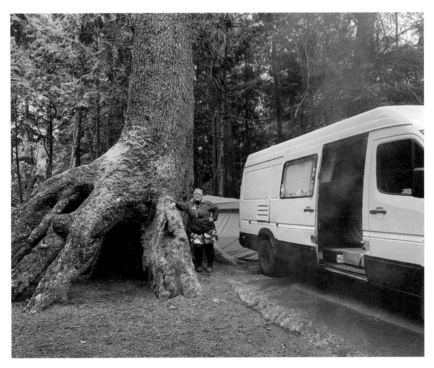

At a campground with my Sprinter van, Towanda, in 2020

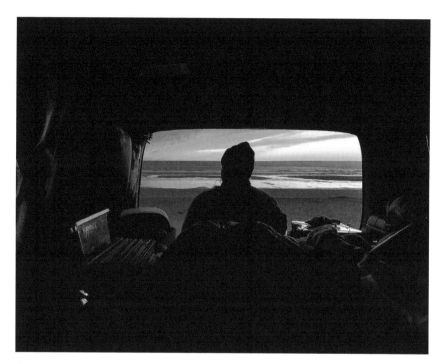

Sunset at the ocean

When I started living in a van, I became, from the outside, the embodiment of stranger danger. From the rust to the horrible peeling paint job to the dark windows, my van was the kind we were warned against as children—"scary" looking. People make assumptions about the person inside the shitty-looking van. I liked that people would see my van and think some dangerous undesirable lived inside. This stereotype kept me safe, because people wouldn't bother me as much. But I have had the police called on me multiple times, and that is never a good experience.

In actuality, I'm a chatty, friendly person. Now that I've lived in one town awhile, more people know who's in that shitty-looking van that's always parked by the ocean. I am an open book, and I never want to have to change that about myself. People often frame trust like it's a thing to be earned, but I like being open. I don't want the trusting aspect of my personality to make me vulnerable or unsafe. Maybe I can be too trusting.

I have had questionably unsafe situations while living in my van. Once, I was in a small town in central Oregon, hiking and checking out the area, and I stopped at a local brewery (one of my favorite things to do when traveling) to get some food and a beer. Being the friendly person that I am, I started chatting with two men at the bar. We talked about Portland and found we had some things in common. Then the tricky question, *Where do you live?*

I'm not always sure if I should answer that question honestly. I feel out each situation, gauge my safety in relation to the person I'm talking to, and follow my intuition. In living openly myself, I tend to think everyone has good intentions. But that doesn't always end up being true.

The men were friendly enough, so I told them about my van life and even showed one of them the inside of my van because he was interested in the lifestyle. He said he liked my setup and admired what I was doing. A beer later though, his friend started talking about a place I used to DJ in Portland and how the "gay people" ruined it. Ugh, here we go. Fuck, why had I trusted this dude? He saw the inside of my van.

He was likely drunk at this point and the female bartender kept locking eyes with me. In the nicest *fuck you* I could mutter, I told him how gay people had, in fact, made that business successful. We exchanged a few more rounds of this before I just didn't feel safe as a gay person, in a small town with no cell service, who was going to sleep in a van that these men had seen. So I paid my tab and started driving. This remote part of Oregon doesn't have many towns, and I ended up driving two hours out of my way, almost running out of gas to get far away from these men and their homophobia. I finally felt safe enough at a campground next to the Deschutes River, tucked behind the trees and shrubbery, with cell service.

Van life is serendipitous, full of unexpected challenges, creative problem solving, adventure, and joy. I love being outside all day, meeting new people, and having a lot of time alone to read, write, reflect, draw, and listen to music. But my favorite part of van life is the way it challenges the status quo. It's rebellious to say, *I don't want to work forty hours at a job just to pay rent.*

Rent has always been the bill I hate most. Why is it so expensive? In Portland, the swiftly rising rents reminded me that my wages had been the same for ten years. And I loved my job before I started living in a van. I was a nanny for seventeen years, and I found it very rewarding. But by the time over half my pay was going to rent, I had realized I no longer belonged in the city. In the land of concrete, ironic, overpriced faux-dive bars, vacant lots becoming condos bought by out-of-state people who work at tech startups, and traffic. It had gotten so bad. It was no longer the place for me. I couldn't keep doing the same things and expect to be fulfilled and happy.

I need dusty gravel back roads at dusk. I need to wave to my neighbors. I need small-town gossip. I need wide open spaces, ok? The Chicks said it first, but I need it too. So, when my girlfriend at the time asked me to move to her small town and live with her and also be a nanny to her kid, I jumped at the opportunity. I was ready for small-town life.

What I didn't realize until it was too late, was that this arrangement isolated me both physically and financially. Soon after the move, she unleashed a full range of narcissistic abuse. It was awful. I became a shell of myself, crying every day, unsure of who I was. I wanted to disappear. And I was confused about how abuse like that could happen to me. I thought I was a strong, independent, smart woman. How did I get here? Van life offered an escape. I couldn't think of any other way to get out of that situation.

While I plotted my escape, I grappled with how to feel safe in my own home. The Safety Kids didn't cover lessons on what to do when you have an abuser in your own bed. When my girlfriend was out of town, I made my getaway plan. I started a fundraiser. I planned a road trip to open FGH chapters across the country and live in my car (and eventually my mom's old minivan). I was desperate. I had to find a way to feel safe again.

Out on the road, far away from the abuse, I found much of the strength I'd forgotten I had. The resilience and joy I pride myself on slowly returned. But I wasn't sure how to heal from the emotional and psychological torment. After leaving her, I would often overreact to small

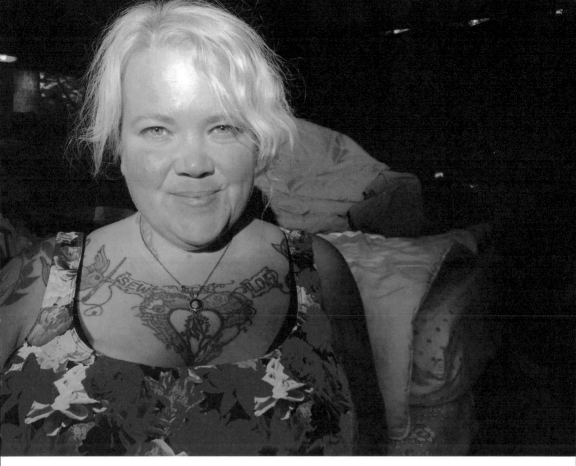

Watching the ocean waves from my previous van, Luna

situations that felt unsafe, becoming panicked. My anxiety and chronic pain soared.

One night, on the side of a mountain overlooking the ocean, where I'd been parking my van overnight for nine months, I lay awake in the dark for hours, quietly listening, convinced I was going to be attacked, thinking I heard footsteps in the gravel outside.

Was I being paranoid? I don't know. Maybe. The fear is real regardless. The truth is, the abuse I survived made me question and doubt every single thing I did. My abuser planted the seed of worthlessness in me. I watered it with self-doubt. I let that shit grow like vines around my heart. And my abuser swung from the branches of her own trauma to laugh in the face of the cyclical pain she inflicted on me.

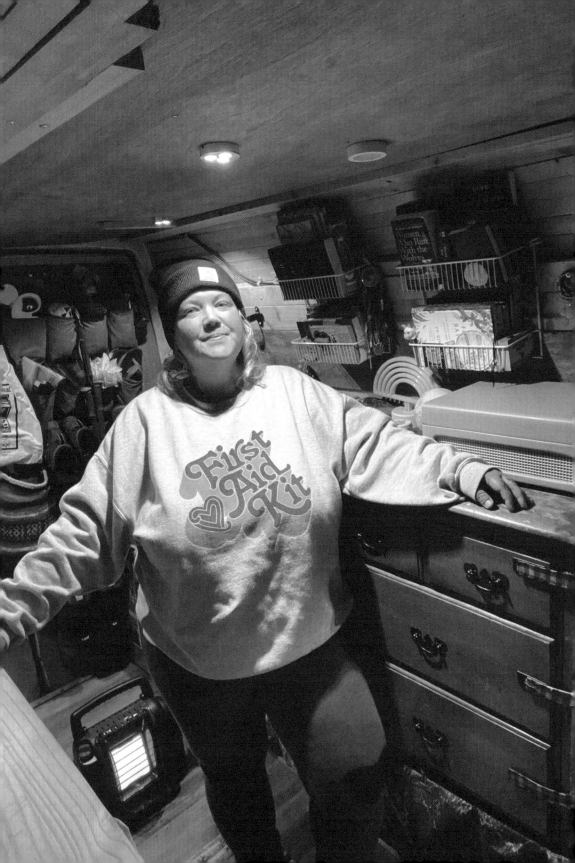

As I heal, I have to honor my instincts. Every time something feels off, I have to really look at it. Instead of brushing off a red flag, I have to trust myself to confront it. I know how to take care of myself and pride myself on being independent. I have strict boundaries that I've developed from all the inner work I've done healing past traumas.

The morning after I spent the night listening for "attackers" outside my van, I cried out all the fear, saying aloud, *You are safe now, you are safe now.* I work every day to actually believe it. How can I ever really be safe if I don't trust myself or listen to my own intuition?

Now, I cultivate an intentional relationship with myself, and I really listen. I have never been happier or more fulfilled in my entire life. I stand up and speak up for myself. I made many choices and endured many setbacks to get to this place of wholeness. My stranger-danger van is gone, replaced by a less "scary"-looking Sprinter van in which I live and write near the Pacific Ocean. Recently, I've been recalling with longing my old apartment in Portland, with its little red desk next to the window that overlooked a schoolyard. But when I look out at the waves as I write, I realize that I have truly made my own dreams come true.

When I was a kid learning about stranger danger, how to stay safe, and what to do if something unsafe happened, I wasn't prepared for what my life would become. I was used to dreaming, but I wasn't used to my dreams coming true. I always wanted this van life by the ocean. Dangerous or not. Since I was a kid, I've always wanted to do things differently than others. It's a peaceful and joyous place to be. I feel content. I have finally found the place that feels like home. I still pinch myself because I cannot believe how happy I feel almost every single day. Which is not to say there aren't challenges or bad days. Every day I make the choice to show up in my life. Every day I make the choice to be outside sitting next to my van with a book, or with my feet in the ocean, or with my boots on a trail, or, on bad chronic pain days, looking at nature from bed. Most of all, though, I feel like I'm really living. I cultivated a life I dreamed of, with joy at the center of it all. I had no idea that dreams could actually come true.

RAQUEL VALDES

(they/them)

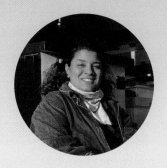

As a kid, I didn't participate in outdoor recreation or camping besides school trips. I was pretty isolated and sheltered. But when I had the chance to be outside, I took it—even if it was just a park in the city, it was a moment to be free and connected with the Earth.

In June 2019, I bought Murphy, a 170 wheelbase diesel Sprinter van. I converted her throughout the hot Sacramento summer and, in October, moved in. I was actually looking to buy a house because I thought, since I was going to be turning thirty soon, that was the next life step I was "supposed" to take. During this time I was in one of my darkest seasons and had made plans to, when I bought my house, leave this realm. Pretty dark, I know. I had to make a choice about what would make me happy. I had dreamt of van life and tiny-home living for years, but it always felt intangible for me specifically—as a person of color, woman of color, and solo traveler, I didn't see myself represented on social media and blogs about that lifestyle.

Though I felt like an outsider when I decided to live in a van instead of a house, I couldn't let it hold me back. Van life saved me from my dark season. I had a will to live, and conquering each day in my van with my dogs and cats has made me the happiest I've ever been. I'm proud that I went for it, claiming my own space in the van life community this past year.

My main purpose in embracing van life is to live tiny and sustainable, and have the opportunity to change my surroundings with a quick drive. I am manic and tend to feel cooped up a lot, but living in the van has really helped because every day I have a new front yard. I try to get outdoors

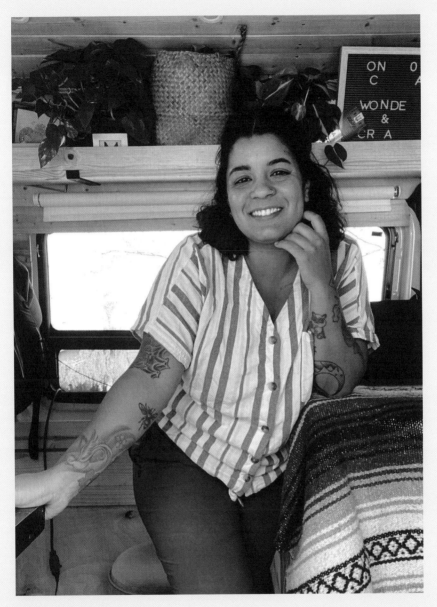

Raquel's van is named Murphy

as often as I can. I set up my office space outside and hangout with the pups. I don't go hiking often, but I do take advantage of any time I can be outside, even if it's for work.

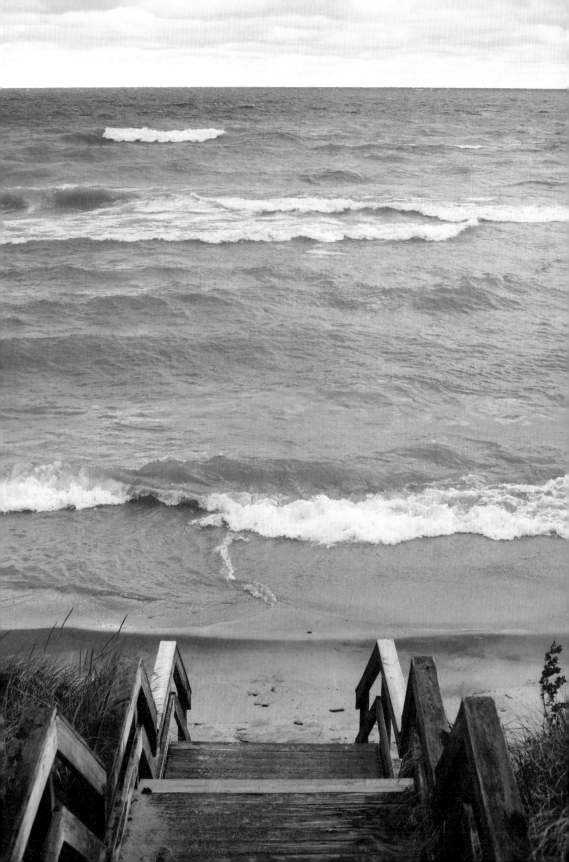

Parking in the forest alongside a river, creek, or lake gives me the best of both worlds, and it's a place I find myself drawn to. My sanity and mental health inspire me to get outside—there I feel grounded, my head clears, and my mood lifts. However, as a woman of color, I have to be cautious of the areas I travel to. Visiting remote outdoor spaces means driving through small rural towns. I've been shouted at while driving through towns like this. As a safety precaution, I make sure to find a place to park at least an hour away from any places where I've been harassed. I often feel isolated and stressed when traveling because I have to be extra cautious and aware of my surroundings. I try to be as invisible as possible, but I just can't truly enjoy boondocking in rural or remote areas. One of the reasons I do a lot of urban dwelling in cities is so I don't have to worry about harassment. The pandemic has been an added challenge because it has changed my access to showers and WiFi. I used to use cafes as my office to get work done, but now I don't have that luxury.

Social media can be great for meeting people. Whenever I've had issues along my journey and have reached out on my Instagram page, I've received a ton of advice and support from fellow van lifers who are open and willing to help however they can. That is community.

Unfortunately, people who live in vehicles are often looked at as lower class, unless they have a high-end vehicle. Like everything, van life has been gentrified, and anyone who doesn't fit a certain mainstream demographic, appearance, or "look" isn't applauded—thin, non-marginalized people with money are told they are so brave and amazing and are glorified for the van lifestyle. It frustrates me that the mainstream van life community is like this. It took me months to find POC van-lifers on Instagram and YouTube. If more companies and van-life communities would sponsor and share stories of POC and get us involved in more nomad gatherings, we could start to see a broader representation for marginalized people. We won't see change unless we claim the spaces we want to be a part of.

So, go claim space—make it yours.

BADLANDS NATIONAL PARK
SOUTH DAKOTA

Summer Michaud-Skog (she/her)
FGH founder

Upon arrival at Badlands National Park, I went into the Ben Reifel Visitor Center to inquire about the park's ADA-accessible trails and found that, although the park rangers and folks who work in the visitor center have a vast amount of knowledge about the region's geology and wildlife, they were less familiar with ADA-accessible trails. They were able to find a pamphlet behind the visitor center desk, and this helped me find a few gorgeous and ADA-accessible boardwalk trails with benches for resting or marveling at the unique geological formations.

Badlands National Park feels like a different planet. The geological formations are truly awe-inspiring. I came here on a road trip with my family when I was younger, but at the time, I wasn't interested in all the National Park has to offer. Now when I visit, my curiosity about the area's plants, wildlife, and geological history is immense. There is so much to see and learn here. The landscape has a ruggedness that is unique to anywhere I've ever seen.

DISTANCE ROUND TRIP Door Trail is 0.25 miles to the viewing deck; the trail continues but is not ADA accessible beyond the viewing deck. Window Trail is 0.3 miles round trip.

ELEVATION GAIN Door Trail gains 50 feet if you hike the entire thing—if you stop at the viewing deck, elevation gain is minimal. Window Trail gains only 10 feet.

CELL SERVICE No cell service. The Ben Reifel Visitor Center, 2 miles south on Highway 240, has WiFi.

ADA AND GENERAL ACCESSIBILITY Both trails are ADA accessible and can accommodate wheelchairs, mobility devices, and strollers. There are benches along the boardwalk and at the viewing areas.

BATHROOMS Yes. There are two single-stall, all-gender, ADA-accessible bathrooms in the trailhead parking lot.

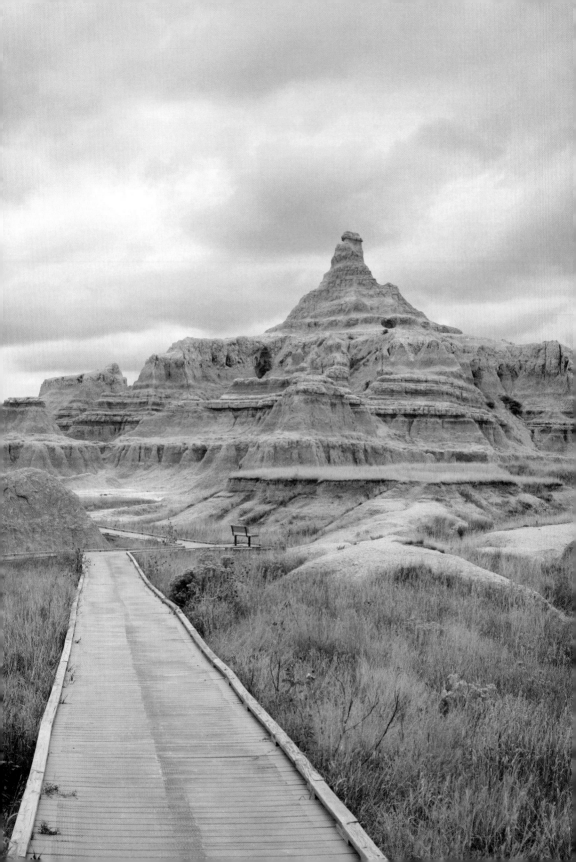

NATIVE LANDS Sioux, Cheyenne, and Lakota. Visit the White River Visitor Center in the South Unit of the park on the Pine Ridge Reservation. It is comanaged by the Oglala Lakota Tribe and offers history, cultural heritage, and information about the area.

TRAIL DESCRIPTION Door and Window Trail are boardwalk trails leading to viewing areas that showcase the dramatic landscape of the Badlands Wall, a 100-mile-long

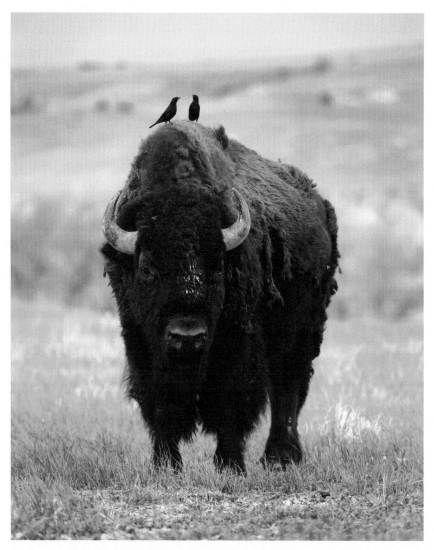

Cowbirds perch on a bison in Badlands National Park in South Dakota

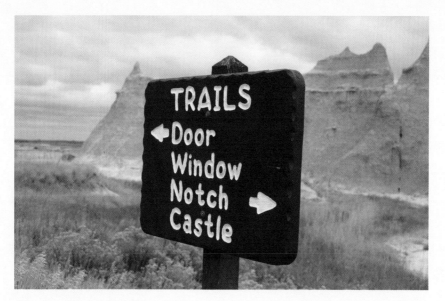

Door and Window Trails sign

ridge made of sandstones, siltstones, mudstones, claystones, limestones, volcanic ash, and shale. Depending on the time of year you visit, you may see wildflowers as well.

OFFICIAL PARK ADDRESS Badlands National Park, Highway 240, Interior, SD 57750

TRAIL NAME Door Trail and Window Trail

HOW TO FIND THE TRAILHEAD From Ben Reifel Visitor Center, travel approximately 2 miles north on Highway 240. The trailhead for both Door and Window Trails are connected by the same parking lot. Look for signs on the east side of the highway. There is no fee to access these trails, but other areas of the National Park do require a parking permit.

SUMMER'S HIKING TIPS Stay on the designated trails to protect this beautiful and fragile natural environment. Take the scenic route on Highway 240 through the National Park. There are many places to pull over and view the scenery. Typically, you can see black-tailed prairie dogs, mule deer, pronghorn (commonly called antelope), bison, coyotes, and bighorn sheep right from your vehicle. Respect the land and the animals here, keep your distance, and pack out everything you bring into the park.

JUPITER

(they/them)

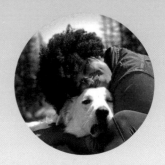

I started van life (actually, not-van life) officially in July 2020. In August 2019, I purchased a 1979 Coachmen Leprechaun camper and started the build for my rig. I was genuinely tired of paying into a system that doesn't benefit me, specifically rent. I named the rig Hot Dog (Hottie for short).

At first I started out with the not-van life idea to see how much better I could do on a test like the LSAT if I spent my time traveling and living rent-free with minimal stressors. Then, it became this sort of exercise in Black joy as a praxis of liberation. I'd paid off my student loans and wanted to feel more secure in my housing situation and more inspired by my work. At the time, I planned to renovate the rig to study for the LSAT so I could attend law school, but Covid put those plans on hold and now I'm just enjoying the experience of a joyful life.

One of the most challenging aspects of van life has been mechanical issues. They're expensive and, eleven out of ten times, also inconvenient. I started my journey with Hottie doing the stoplight shuffle (swiftly putting her in park every stop) and now she runs like a dream. But so much happened in between—from fires to three weeks off the road so she could get a new carburetor. It's been tough, but I've learned so much along the way.

I have been on an incredible journey working to build a world that ensures other people can access and tap into their own joy in the ways I've been so fortunate to do. It feels like this work is a big part of the purpose behind why I live the way I do—maybe it's the whole thing. Currently I'm funemployed. I freelance write and that's basically how I make my

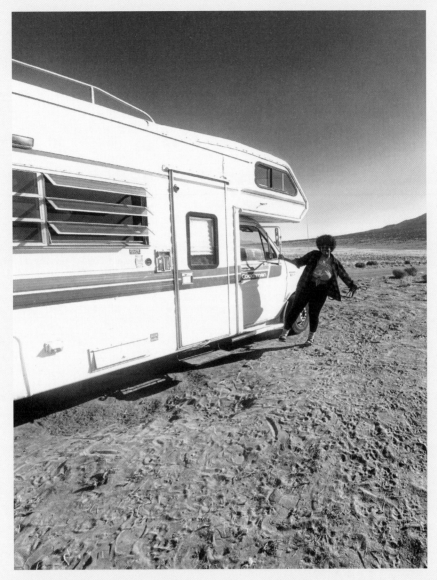

Jupiter with their home-on-wheels, Hottie

income. I write about subjects I'm passionate about like social justice, racial equity, and prison abolition advocacy.

As a kid, I rode dirt bikes and went camping. I had a tree house in my backyard and a couple dogs I was never without. We didn't have a lot of

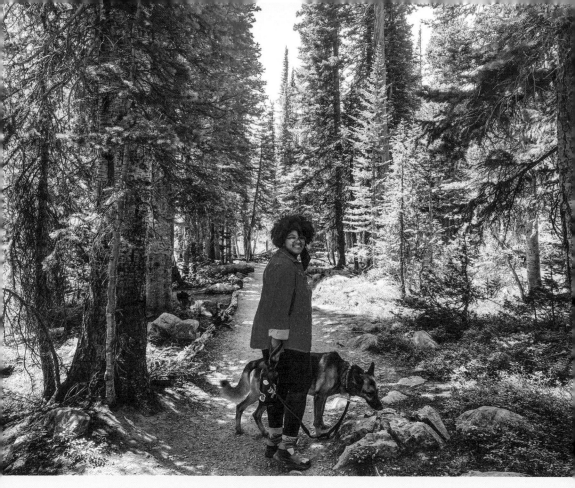

Jupiter takes time outside with one of their dogs

money, so going outside was my activity of choice. I've been hooked since. I have always enjoyed being outdoors. I like quiet and solitude, and outside has always had more than its fair share of both. I do yoga outside in the morning and on working days I try to spend most, if not all, of my day outside.

I've been very fond of the mountains lately, but I'm really truly a beach being at heart. I adore the sounds of the waves, the salty breeze, spending entire days in the ocean, and of course the sunshine.

Now that we live on the road, I know my dogs love our increased outdoor time. I love my time with them and want to make sure they're living their best lives. I'm also getting really into outdoor photography, and I think the excitement of going outside armed with a camera makes exploring just that much better.

When you become interested in new activities, it can be intimidating when you don't see anyone that looks like you—but it's even worse when you confront people about the lack of representation and they give an answer along the lines of, *well, Black people just don't do XYZ*. This is, of course, almost entirely false. Black people are outside. Black people hike. We swim, we climb, we take photos outdoors, and many of us truly thrive in spaces white people have managed to convince themselves exist only for their benefit. That's as true for rock climbing and nature photography as it is of living in a rig.

The culture around van life is as steeped in racism as the outdoor industry. A whitewashed, cishetero, able-bodied, endlessly picturesque image of van life has been built up and reinforced by the van-life community for years. It doesn't help at all that the initial buy-in costs to start van life can be prohibitive to folks from systematically oppressed communities. When these barriers combine, it becomes very easy—in fact, sometimes it still happens to me—to believe that these spaces just weren't meant for us to enjoy or thrive in. I'm very privileged that right now, in addition to trying to figure out how to afford surprise mechanic visits, these are the most pressing barriers to my life outdoors and on the road. I've typically got enough saved that I can handle whatever Hottie throws at me whether I like it or not. And I'm never at a loss for a place to shower or cry about whatever needs to be repaired next.

I've also been relatively lucky that I've not experienced much bigotry on the road. This is likely to due with the fact that the pandemic hit shortly after I started my not-van life, which limited my interactions with other outdoor folks. However, there was one specific incident where my partner and I were driving through rural Colorado and had to choose between gas (when both of our tanks were on E) and our personal safety. The only gas station within thirty miles was swamped with white supremacist supporters waving terrible flags and yelling at passersby. Luckily, we made it to the next gas station, but it was a close call.

Van life communities need to be more intentional about the ways in which marginalized individuals and voices are shared. When mainstream van life accounts participate in things like #PassTheMic (in which larger van-life accounts and community pages temporarily hand over access to their audience to a Black van lifer with less reach), they have to be sincere in their efforts and acknowledge that it must be an ongoing effort to diversify those they choose to represent on their social media pages. Otherwise, Black people become tokens and filler for the further promotion of a brand that doesn't actually include us. This year saw many online campaigns claiming to want to diversify van life, but once Black lives stopped being trendy, things went right back to business as usual with less representation and Black lives only mattering when Black lives are lost. It's hard to want to use products or join hiking groups or go climb with folks who see you as a trend or a bonus instead of as a person.

I didn't feel like I had a sense of community when I was living in an apartment, but now that I'm part of this large group of folks who live in vans, buses, and RVs, I do. I'm so grateful to be able to help cultivate this community with these folks. It's important to have people in my life who understand the random stuff that happens on the road. Shared experiences and similar interests have brought me close to people I might have never known otherwise, and now we have the opportunity to grow together. I'm pretty new at navigating van life as a Black, non-binary individual, but the community I have found is everything.

When I got on the road the first time, it was the most joyous experience I've had in my not-van. Despite all the quirks and hardships, a sense of accomplishment overwhelmed me—I had sat myself down and said I was gonna build out a camper, and I had actually done it. I hit the road to live out my dreams. It's just me, my dogs, my rig, and the open road, with nothing to do but exist and pursue whatever sets my soul on fire.

Every lifestyle is tough in its own way. Van life is one of the most amazing and flexible choices you can make. People feel like apartment life isn't for them all the time, yet they cling to it because that's seen as normal and safe. Once you reject the idea that paying rent or a mortgage symbolizes

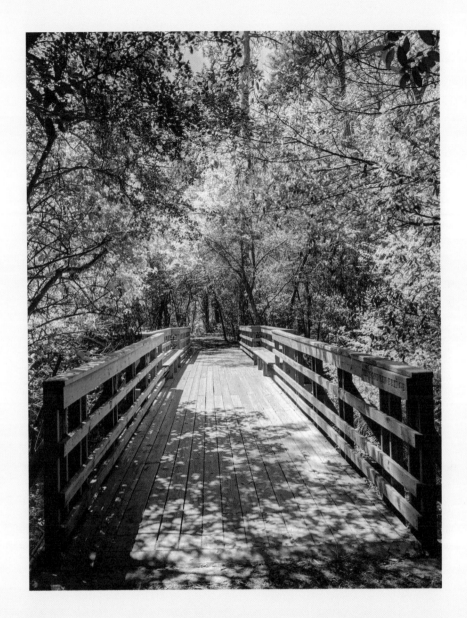

success, you're halfway there. Don't be discouraged if you don't see many people that look like you out there doing it (especially not in mainstream communities). Just get out there. Make mistakes, make art, get lost, take a hike, and have fun.

INWOOD HILL PARK
MANHATTAN, NEW YORK

Vanessa Chica Ferreira (she/her)
FGH chapter: New York, New York

When I was a child, Inwood Hill Park provided an escape for everyone in my neighborhood, a mini vacation from the routine. At any given time, I could watch baseball players set up for a game, sunbathers spread out like daisies, or tired mothers resting while their children played.

I spent years of my childhood here, playing handball, rolling down hills, visiting the nature center, admiring the expansive salt marsh, and exploring the trails where

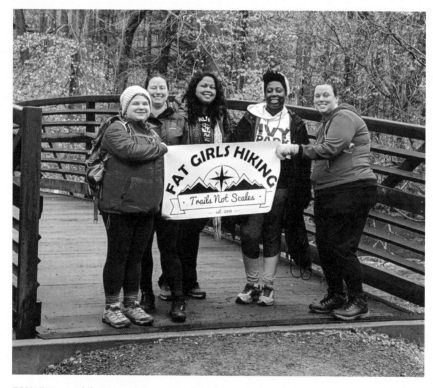

FGH NYC group hike

artifacts from religious offerings were left behind.

I believed I had explored every inch of Inwood, until, as an ambassador for Fat Girls Hiking, I discovered a new trail. There were rock formations I'd never seen and steep hills I'd never climbed. We hiked casually and in conversation. When we were done, we went to a local store to have lemonade.

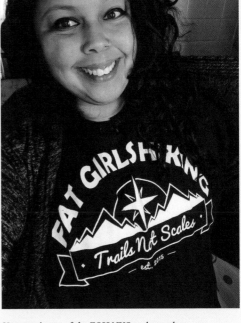

Vanessa is one of the FGH NYC ambassadors

DISTANCE ROUND TRIP 1.3 miles

ELEVATION GAIN 282 feet

CELL SERVICE Yes

ADA AND GENERAL ACCESSIBILITY The Orange Trail is not ADA accessible but other trails in the park are. There are benches throughout the park but not alongside this trail.

BATHROOMS Yes. There are gendered ADA-accessible bathrooms near the trailhead.

NATIVE LANDS Munsee Lenape and Wappinger

TRAIL DESCRIPTION The Orange Trail is a moderate-to-vigorous hike on unpaved paths through the heart of the park's Forever Wild forest, where you can see tulip trees, oaks, and maples.

OFFICIAL PARK ADDRESS Inwood Hill Park, Payson Ave and Seaman Ave, New York, NY 10034

TRAIL NAME Orange Trail

HOW TO FIND THE TRAILHEAD The trailhead is on Dyckman Street and can be found on Google Maps. There's plenty of street parking nearby.

VANESSA'S HIKING TIPS Take your time. Listen to your body. The end of the trail is where you want it to be—you can always turn back. Be kind to your fellow hiking partners. Take the time to build connections and community while you enjoy nature. Have lemonade after, it's optional, but delicious.

FAT ACTIVISM ONLINE

_

BIGOTS, BULLSHIT, AND BOUNDARIES

love the way social media connects us. I can stay in touch with people from around the world. I can stay up to date on people's lives, events, and communities in a super convenient and easy way. I love to share what I'm doing, what I think, beautiful places where I hike, or spots I travel to in my van-home. I love to share other people's art and poetry, rad stuff other folks are doing, and inclusive fat spaces online or in real life that I think my community will want to know about.

My work through Fat Girls Hiking has created an amazing worldwide community and, in turn, created my dream job—all through social media. But, of course, social media has a real dark side. Comparison, trolling, and bullying are prevalent. The frameworks make it almost impossible be the multi-faceted human you are in real life. Feeds are highlight reels of peoples' lives—filled with the most beautiful, curated photos and perfect, meaningful captions—inauthentic or, honestly, fake. You know nobody's life is as flawless as those filters make it look.

Worse though, is that even just existing online as an outdoorsy, fat, queer femme makes me a target for unwarranted advice, harassment, and bullying.

Our culture is built on systems that perpetuate white supremacy, capitalism, colonialism, sexism, and heteronormativity, all of which inform our relationship to our bodies. It's a culture that keeps certain demographics powerful through the oppression of others. Social media reflects aspects of the world we live in. I want to create a space within it where I feel included and seen—a place where I feel I belong.

When Fat Girls Hiking started in 2015, it was mostly about my own hikes and sharing my favorite places to be outdoors. Very early on, I had to defend my right to use the word *fat* to identify myself. People wanted me to use an easier word. But I like identifying as fat. It feels radical. I've always marched to my own beat, so I wasn't too surprised when I found myself passed over many times for articles, collaborations, and paid sponsorships. (Thankfully, using *fat* as a reclamation has become more common and accepted.)

Though I refused to change the FGH name, I would often soften it by using the more inclusive *body positive*. This was a term that had grown out of communities created by and for fat folks. Unfortunately, the more mainstream the body-positive movement became, the more the fat queer women and fat Black women who started the movement

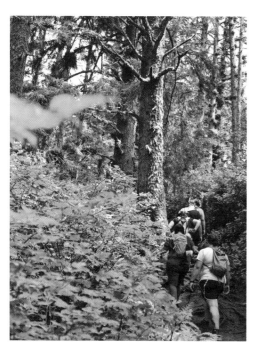

Group hike at Cape Lookout on the Oregon coast

found themselves marginalized and silenced. Taken over by people using it as a profit-focused marketing ploy, body positivity was increasingly represented as thin, white, heterosexual, cisgendered women in yoga pants who wanted to love the roll their stomachs made when they leaned to the side. (Which they should! Love your body, whatever it is.) Diet culture hopped on the body-positivity train and was sold to fat people as "wellness." The language we'd created in our safer community had been co-opted to sell diet culture in a new package.

As my politics grew more radical, I cared less and less about corporations or magazines acknowledging my work—it's the community and all the people in it who motivate me, and I'm fiercely protective of them. I eventually stopped using the term *body positive* because I didn't like the implication that I, or anyone else who lives in a fat or marginalized body, had to be positive about being widely oppressed.

In the beginning, some people thought Fat Girls Hiking was a motivational group for people to lose weight. And since body positivity and self-love had increased traction in the mainstream as part of a pro-diet and weight-loss agenda, I had to again adjust the language around what Fat Girls Hiking is and what it is not. I created community guidelines so anyone attending an event or group hike or participating in the community online could engage in a way that would be best for the care of the community. Fat Girls Hiking doesn't allow diet or weight-loss talk. We also don't allow racism, sexism, homophobia, transphobia, classism, ableism, or any form of bigotry. These guidelines are now part of our mission statement, which I constantly post about (every hike and event description includes them) because social media often feels like a never-ending battle against anti-fat diet-culture trolls.

Interrupting diet talk is exhausting, y'all. I found myself continually justifying my right to simply exist as a fat person who wanted to hike with other fat and marginalized people and allies. *Why do we need all these separate groups for people hiking? If you want to hike, just go hike. You're just dividing people more by separating yourselves into a different group.** I had to fight relentlessly when people wanted to say homophobic things about me as a queer woman because they wanted this community to just be about fat girls hiking. *You made the group uncomfortable when you said you were queer. No one was there looking for a date.**

Over time, I adjusted the FGH guidelines through my experiences to curate the space I wanted to thrive in and offer to others. My goal is online and real-life spaces and communities where we can all be fully who we are without shame or justification or explanation. Initially, I made the

*actual things people have messaged to me

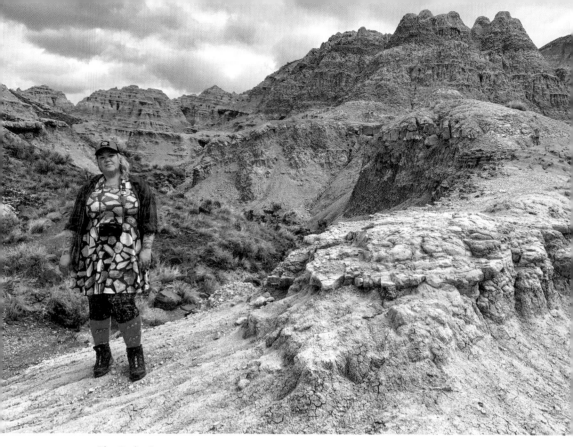

Blue Basin, Oregon

mistake of saying all were welcome. But that's not actually true. I won't welcome bigots into this community. If someone is bothered by the fact that I talk not only about being a fat woman in the outdoors but also about being queer, then this community may not be for them. If someone is looking for a place to share how they have lost weight through hiking a lot, this is not the community for them. People can do whatever they want with their bodies and participate or not in diet and weight-loss culture, but in this tiny microcosm on the internet, I won't allow it. It's okay though—there are literally thousands of places online and IRL where you can talk about diet culture. It's everywhere.

In order to keep the online FGH space free from diet culture, weight-loss talk, body shaming, and any form of bigotry, I had to invest time in creating language and tactics for when trolls or anyone else comes into the space without respect for the guidelines. As the community has grown, so have the bigoted and misinformed emails, messages, and comments from strangers.

Online trolls come into community spaces intended for marginalized folks, spout their opinions, and say it's their right because of freedom of speech. Trolls are people who hide behind keyboards and give weight-loss advice in spaces that have anti-diet guidelines. Trolls are strangers who message my friends about how I'm problematic because I have strict online boundaries.

Imagine if people read the stuff I wrote and instead of having a knee-jerk reaction about how I'm "promoting obesity" because I love my fat body, they just kept scrolling or unfollowed me. Try it. It's absolutely liberating to realize you are, in a lot of ways, in control of what you see on your social media feed. *Unfollow* and *block* are your self-care friends.

I readily block people who exhibit toxic behaviors. I unfollow people who post content that makes me feel like shit. I don't have to justify why I block someone. I have the right to protect my emotional energy, what I'm exposed to, and who can direct ideas my way.

Many people doing social justice work are, like me, burned out by the constant, free emotional labor that comes with speaking out against oppression. It happens to almost every activist I know online. Imagine the things we could do with our time if we didn't have to deal with this.

For a long time, I didn't use my last name when writing articles or being interviewed by journalists about Fat Girls Hiking. I feared the backlash of anti-fat health-concern trolls, bigots, and bullies. I stopped accepting direct messages on Facebook because I didn't want to deal with hateful messages anymore. I no longer have a direct email link on the FGH website because of the immense number of messages it was receiving from people who wanted to shame or harm me. I still fear the trolls and the bullies, but I'm not willing to hide my true self from the community I've built.

I go through cycles of loving my work and having a hard time remembering why I do it. I do it because I love this community—its members are constantly lifting me up and supporting the work I do to create a vision of the outdoors in which they see themselves represented. I am inspired by the people I message with who are finding their way out of diet culture and want to heal in the outdoors with others. I can't do this work alone. When I feel isolated, I always want to share and be vulnerable with the community. When messages from trolls make me cry, I want y'all to know, because your messages of support keep me going.

I've had people tell me that the work I'm doing changed their life. I even got a message once from someone who said I *saved* her life. This is powerful and meaningful. I am here for it. How can one toxic message from someone I don't know make that disappear? I tell myself that the work I do is important. I tell myself that it's okay to struggle. I tell myself that though this work might sometimes exhaust and challenge me, I will do my best to believe in myself fully. It's a practice, not a destination. It changes and fluctuates. I continue to grow and develop as a more kind, accepting, open, and vulnerable human, regardless of what some may say or think about me or the work I do.

It's easy to believe people when they say things about me that I fear might be true even though I know they really aren't. I'm a recovering people pleaser. I have lived my whole life helping people. As an older sibling in a family of five with a single mom who worked multiple jobs to make ends meet, I always wanted to ease her burdens. I helped by caring for my younger brothers, cleaning, and cooking. My mom is one of the most amazing humans I've ever known, and I wanted to do anything I could to make her life a little easier, but I was a sensitive kid and teenager and the suffering of others can be a heavy burden. I always wanted to ease others' pain. I still do. People who suffer or have had hard lives or can't see their own amazing qualities, those are the people I'm drawn to.

As a recovering people pleaser, I have learned how to have healthy boundaries (saying no without guilt), how to have balanced relationships and friendships (keeping friends and relationships where I get as much as I give), and that I can block people in real or online life who take advantage of my giving nature, are toxic, or don't respect me.

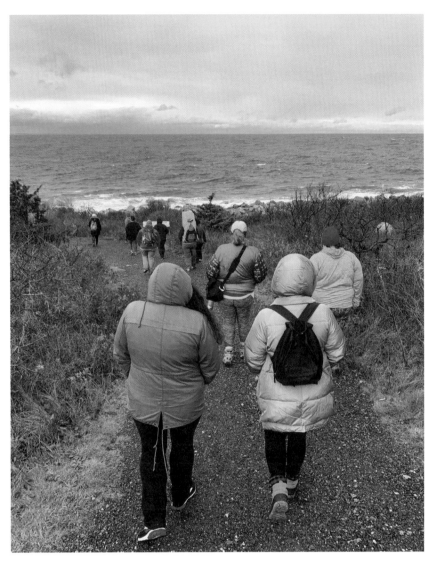

Group hike, Halibut Point State Park, Massachusetts

Being a people pleaser is not only about saying yes when I want to say no—it's also about feeling somehow obligated to say yes. At a young age, media and culture taught me that being good, saying yes, and pleasing people were the only acceptable ways for girls to take up space in this

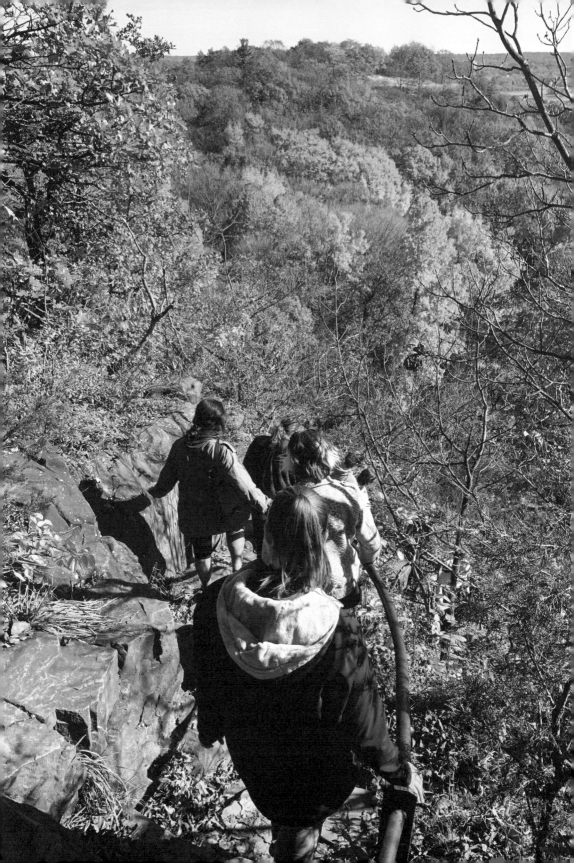

world. I was afraid to be hurt by rejection, so I protected myself by being good. I felt like if I was good and helpful, people would like me. And I wanted to be liked.

It's an unhealthy cycle, and I want to be free from it. The truth is, I can't control what strangers on the internet think about me, see in me, or say about me. And I do my best to remember that it's not my job to be liked. As Mary Oliver's poem *Wild Geese*, reminds me, "You only have to let the soft animal of your body love what it loves."

So, what do I do when trolls get me down?

I reach out. I text my loved ones who know me well. I write. I remember that I am not *only* this work. I am me, a multi-faceted human who is strong, kind, loving, understanding, open, smart, vulnerable, silly, and also insecure, exhausted, self-doubting, imperfect, sad, tired, and always wanting everyone to like me.

All I can do is live my truth and be authentic and vulnerable. I can use my voice and my experience to connect with others who see themselves in the hard times I'm going and have gone through. Remembering I'm not alone validates my experiences. Stories from the lives of other marginalized people, vulnerability, and connection, these are the things I love about social media. We are not alone. Many of you feel this way.

Self-care and community care is very important to me. My current troll policy is to screenshot and report their messages and comments, block, delete, and share publicly. Responding to people who approach my work with the intent to be "right" about how fat people are wrong for speaking up about anti-fatness, oppression, weight stigma, and diet culture is an incredibly draining distraction. If people are trying to understand my stance on something or want to ask a question, I now know that I don't have to respond. I don't have to be good, pleasing, or be liked by everyone. I have the right to not respond. I have the right to protect my energy, time, and well-being. I don't owe strangers on the internet anything (and neither do you!). I don't have the capacity for it anymore because I'm too busy changing and saving peoples' lives.

SAM ORTIZ

(she/her)

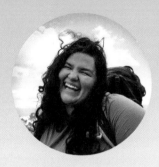

The drama of mountains, with their jagged edges, unforgiving slopes, and ever-changing weather, has always spoken to me in a way that no other landscape does. The mountains teach me so many of life's lessons: how the smallest of steps put together can carry me incredible lengths; how small I am in the bigness of it all; and how to understand that everything is interconnected. Mountains motivate me, especially when I can look back and see how far I've come. They prove to me that I am strong. They show me that hard things are so often worth it. And, perhaps most importantly, they show me that hard things get easier over time and with practice.

I grew up in Kentucky near the Red River Gorge, on the ancestral land of the Osage, Cherokee, Shawandasse Tula, S'atsoyaha, Adena, and Hopewell people. The gorge is a world-class rock-climbing destination, and though I'd spent some time there hiking, whenever I was invited to go rock climbing, I always said no. When I look back now, I know why I turned those invitations down—I didn't see myself in any of the people recreating there. I saw very few people of color, and I never once saw a fat person climbing. I simply didn't think a person like me could do something like that. I've always loved the outdoors, but I haven't always felt permission to take up space there. It wasn't until many years after I moved away from the Red River Gorge that I finally felt permission to attempt something as scary as rock climbing, and it was because of the people who offered to mentor me and help me learn along the way.

When I moved to Juneau, Alaska, after college, I desperately wanted to drink in the magic of the mountains, but I didn't know how or where to start hiking. For anyone who didn't grow up in the outdoors, entering the great unknown can be really overwhelming and intimidating. I had someone to walk me through it, which made all the difference. It was there, in the ancestral land of the Tlingit and Dënéndeh people, that I finally found the courage to start taking up space. Each day I spent immersed in nature, I learned more about myself and felt more drawn to break down my own expectations about who I was destined to become.

There is one single day that I credit as the pivotal point of my life. It was the last week of my time living in Juneau, and I decided to attempt a feat that I felt I couldn't complete—hiking to the summit of Mount Juneau. I knew I would go very slowly. I knew I would take breaks. I fully expected to fail. But I also knew that it was my last chance to try. After many breaks and many moments spent questioning whether or not I could continue, I made it to the top. Completing a six-mile hike might not be a huge accomplishment for many people, but for me it changed everything.

Hiking Mount Juneau was the first time I let myself try something even though I thought I might fail. Completing this hike taught me that

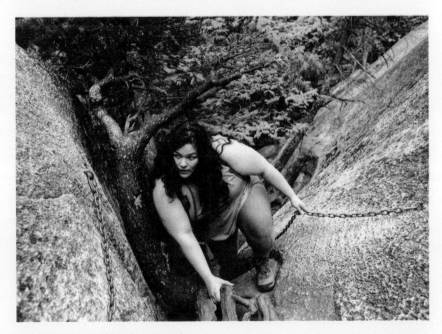

Sam believes you can't be what you can't see

maybe, just maybe, I might not fail at all. It helped me prove to myself that even if something is scary and takes a long time, it's still worth doing. Perhaps most importantly, I taught myself that I am capable of incredible things if I can only get the courage to begin. I've carried the lessons I learned about myself on Mount Juneau with me and used them to inform my decisions ever since.

When I decided to stop letting the fear of failure hold me back from new, hard experiences, I learned pretty quickly that my plus-size body can do some really amazing feats. My body walks up tall, steep mountains. My body carries everything I need to survive in the wilderness on my back for days at a time. My body scales rock walls, even when my hands shake with fear. My body rappels into canyons. My body kayaks and swims and rafts in white water and so many other things.

The outdoors offers me some of the only opportunities in my life that challenge me to appreciate my body and the incredible things it can do for me. It helps me to be present with myself in each moment and present with how my body is feeling and what it needs. When I'm outside, I focus on the amazing things my body is capable of—it feels strong, and I feel confident in my power.

Now when I recreate outdoors, one of my goals is to mentor, teach, and inspire other people. There is an incredible need for community and representation for plus-size people, especially in climbing and outdoor adventure sports. Plus-size bodies are simply not represented in adventure media and are often specifically excluded when it comes to things like technical gear. Fat climbers are even more rarely represented.

The average US woman is a size 16 or higher, yet the gear options available don't represent that. Even though there is a market of people who are willing to buy products, outdoor retailers are often unwilling to have us as customers. Not only do people not expect us to be there but the gatekeepers also actively exclude us from participating. By just showing up in outdoor spaces and participating in adventure activities, I am showing that my body and bodies like mine deserve to be there. My body taking up space in a place where people and institutions have tried to exclude

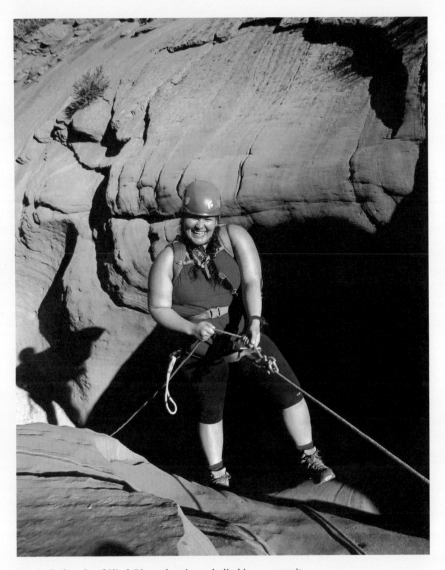

Sam is the founder of Climb Big, a plus-size rock climbing community

me is an act of resistance. Recreation for fat hikers and climbers is an act of resistance.

When I first started climbing I had never seen anyone who looked like me rock climb before. In fact, even after I had been climbing for years,

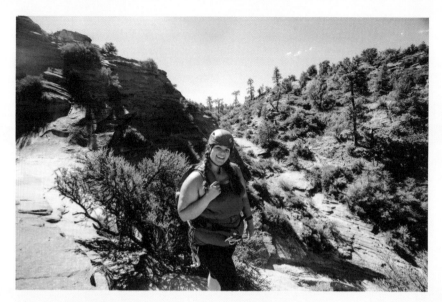

Sam advocates for inclusion for plus-size people in rock climbing

I still struggled to find even a single other plus-size person who could relate to me in the climbing community. Eventually I connected with other badass plus-size climbers online, but still—the handful of people I found didn't feel like enough.

I started hosting plus-size climbing meetups for beginners. Many attendees have told me that a plus-size-specific event is the only way they ever would have considered trying rock climbing. The barriers for plus-size people to get into climbing can feel immense. Worrying about whether the harness will fit (or worse, trying to fit into a harness and not being able to), worrying about whether the rope is strong enough to hold you, and worrying about not being strong enough to pull yourself up are all very real concerns. I've heard those fears from countless folks, and they're the same fears I had all those years ago.

Mentorship is one of the most important and high-leverage opportunities we have to make the outdoors more welcoming and accessible. There is such a wide variety of things to learn before getting started in the outdoors that it can feel incredibly overwhelming. So many people who love nature simply don't know where to begin learning the skills they need to safely recreate outdoors. However when someone has the opportunity for mentorship, so much opens up for them. Not only does it make the outdoors less scary but it also gives them someone to ask questions and learn from.

You can't be what you can't see. Every time I feel scared or too vulnerable to show my body, I think about younger me. I think about how much it would have impacted me if I had seen myself represented in outdoor sports. I think about all the times I said no to something because I felt like I didn't belong or because I was afraid of how I would look. I think about all the times I told myself *you can't* instead of trying. One of my friends challenged me to be the role model that I, myself, needed. That challenge has inspired me to create the things I didn't see in the world.

As a fat rock climber I saw very few other people with similar body types climbing, so I decided to change that. Because I didn't feel like I fit into any particular place within the outdoor community I decided to create the community that I wanted instead. I created Climb Big to help develop a community of fat climbers. What started as just a project about climbing became much larger, however. Many of us didn't realize that we'd never intentionally created space for plus-size friendships before. I know I hadn't. Distinctly calling out and embracing our plus-size bodies has had a power and a visibility. It creates a strength and community that I never knew was missing before.

EDITH L. MOORE NATURE SANCTUARY
HOUSTON, TEXAS

Laura Burns (she/her)
FGH chapter: Houston, Texas

I've always felt a strong connection to the natural world, especially when in water or among trees. To this day, I feel most connected to the earth and free in my body when I'm swimming and hiking. Unfortunately, as a fat kid, teen, and young adult, I learned that my body was less welcome in these spaces and stopped trying to be there as much. At some point though, I decided that I deserve to be on a trail or in the water as much as anyone else. I'm a fat woman, a person of color, and slow as heck on the trail—and that's okay! We all deserve to be there, taking up space and connecting with nature in the bodies we have today. We don't need to wait until we fit a certain image in order to get outside.

The Edith L. Moore Nature Sanctuary is a beautiful natural space right in the city. Though you're near a huge freeway and can sometimes hear a little traffic, it is peaceful and has tons to offer. The trail is teeming with all kinds of birds that sing constantly. Much of the hike is alongside a creek where you can see wildlife and hear the water flowing. Before or after your hike, it's really fun to visit the historic cabin and see the history of the building and property. There are also ponds and a nursery that grows native plants.

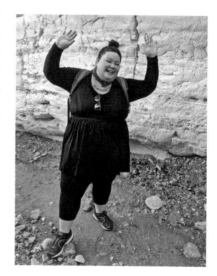

Laura is a fierce, fat, feminist who loves connecting to nature

The FGH Houston chapter came here for our second group hike. We had a group of about ten and hiked slowly around the trail, learning about the types of trees and birds found in the sanctuary (it's a big list). We stopped behind the

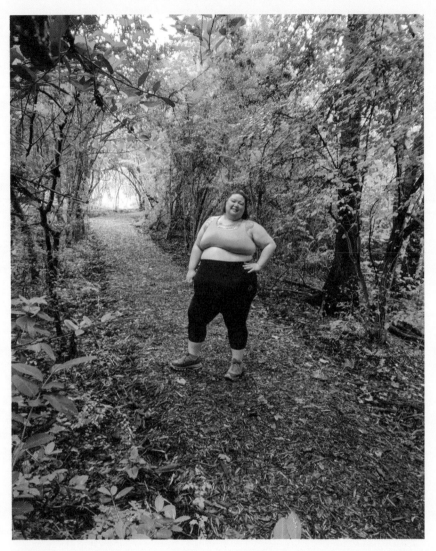

A yoga instructor, Laura created Radical Body Love Yoga to help people find the healing benefits of yoga and body liberation

historic cabin and practiced some gentle accessible yoga and enjoyed the day together. It was a beautiful moment, and we felt so connected and strong as a community. While we were lingering, trying to spot turtles in the pond, we decided to make them our mascot. Now on group hikes, we look for (and usually find) a turtle or two to snap a selfie with.

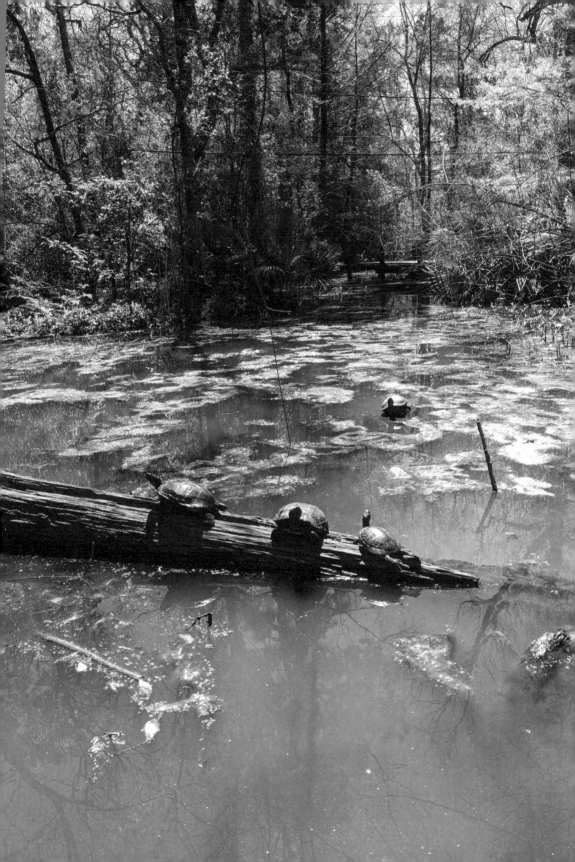

DISTANCE ROUND TRIP 1.5 miles

ELEVATION GAIN 20 feet

CELL SERVICE Yes

ADA AND GENERAL ACCESSIBILITY The trail is not ADA accessible, though most of it is passable for wheelchairs, mobility devices, and strollers. There are a few areas with elevation gain and loss that aren't accessible, but it's easy to bypass them. There are a few benches along the trail where you can rest, but they're mostly located toward the beginning and end and not in the middle.

BATHROOMS Sometimes. There are bathrooms onsite in the historic cabin, however they're only open when staff is on the premises and those hours are not dependable. Nearby businesses also have bathrooms.

NATIVE LANDS Coahuiltecan, Karankawa, and Sana

TRAIL DESCRIPTION This shady forest trail in West Houston is part of the 17.5–acre wooded preserve along Rummel Creek. There's an educational center and a self-led trail guide you can use to explore and learn about the history of the site, trees, birds, and other wildlife. The Houston Audubon Society maintains the nature sanctuary, and they've created a stop–by–stop guide you can access on your cell phone. There's only one trail here that runs next to the creek most of the time. It's a lollipop–shaped, soft–dirt and mulch trail with lots of fun bridges and some benches along the way for resting. Stay after your hike to check out the historic cabin, history information, and small ponds with turtles and fish. No dogs are allowed unless you hold a permit.

OFFICIAL PARK ADDRESS Edith L. Moore Nature Sanctuary, 440 Wilchester Blvd, Houston, TX 77079

TRAIL NAME The self-guided trail system comprises lots of little trails strung together to form a choose–your–own–adventure loop. You'll start out on the Mary Cravens Trail or the West Bank Trail, which soon connect.

HOW TO FIND THE TRAILHEAD The entrance to the nature sanctuary is on a residential street that offers some parking, and Huston Audubon recommends parking in at the Memorial Methodist Church. The trailhead is right by the historic cabin and is easy to find.

KRISTIE BRINGHURST

(she/her)

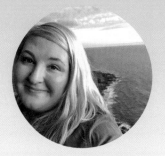

When I was very little, around eight years old, I liked being outside. This lasted until I was made aware that my body should be thinner. Then I spent more and more time inside and isolated, where I could ignore my body and watch TV instead.

When I was a teenager, I went hiking for a church activity, and it was much steeper and muddier than the counselors had expected. Despite the fact that I was an active teen—I played basketball and volleyball—I struggled while my friends did not. They hiked ahead, having conversations I couldn't be a part of as I struggled at the back. I blamed myself and vowed I would never hike again. Looking back, I'm sad that I blamed myself, and I'm glad that my perspective has changed.

The word *hiking* has always been scary to me. I thought it meant traversing mountains—not something I felt I could do. It wasn't until about three years ago, when I started participating in an inclusive outdoor community, that I started to understand *hiking* means spending time outdoors, and that it can be as hard or as easy as I want it to be. It's about nature, it's not about my ability.

A couple months ago, I had a doctor's appointment at which I was terribly fat-shamed and the doctor refused to treat me. My partner came to get me and we drove to Collins Beach just outside Portland on a Wednesday afternoon. We walked along the beach and waded in the water freely with no one else around. The sun was shining and the cool water was lapping against my shins. I felt perfectly at peace and connected to the earth. It helped me heal.

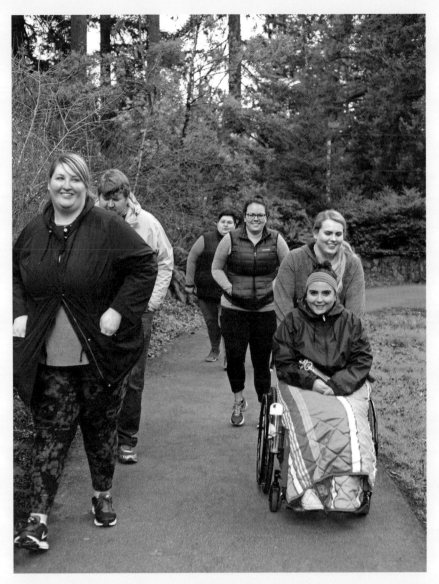

Kristie has found an inclusive outdoor community where she can show up as she is

To be honest, I still struggle with outdoor recreation because it can feel scary to do it on my own. That's why outdoor community is so important to me. The outdoors doesn't feel quite so intimidating when I'm with others who accept me. With my chronic pain, walking far can

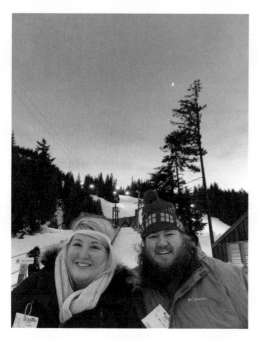

Kristie and her husband on a FGH adventure in Oregon

be difficult. There are so few trails or parks that have benches or smooth terrain, so it can be tricky choosing a place to hike. I also fear judgment and public call-outs when I'm outside and have to take frequent breaks.

I think for me, most of the bigotry I've faced in the outdoors has been from my own internal anti-fatness. When I was young and would go for the rare hike with friends, my brain would constantly be on a loop, saying terrible things to myself and worrying about how red my face was as I tried to limit my breathing so my exertion wouldn't be noticed or criticized. The biggest bigotry I've experienced from other people is when we're supposed to be hiking together but they refuse to slow down or wait for me to catch up. It's punishing.

As someone who is size 32, about 5X, I have begun to find pants suitable for wearing outdoors in my size. However, it's virtually impossible for me to find a breathable jacket or raincoat I can wear hiking. Very few companies carry plus sizes and if they do, they only carry what are considered "acceptable" plus sizes, which stop at 2X or 3X. The outdoor industry is exclusionary by nature. Pun intended. That's why extended size ranges are so important. I want to see the outdoor industry offer 6X and beyond, possibly even custom sizing. I also want to see them using a range of plus-size models, models in wheelchairs, nonbinary models, and people of color. Right now, outdoor recreation is tailored for thin, white, able-bodied people, and the industry (outfitters, gear companies, equipment brands) keeps it that way when they don't offer sizes for plus-size people and expansive representation. One symptom of this is that some thin people have a weird possessiveness toward the outdoors—when I show up, it's as if I've trespassed on their territory.

An inclusive outdoor community was one of the main reasons I moved to Oregon from Salt Lake City, which, although it is known for fitness and hiking, did not offer me a safe community with whom to experience the outdoors. At my first FGH event, I was a little scared and dealing with some back pain. On the hike to Wahclella Falls, I began to struggle, and a member of the group turned around and offered me the trekking poles she was using. I remember being taken aback that someone would do that for me. The poles made the hike easier, and I felt supported and comforted, not just by the equipment but by that hiker and also by the hike leader, who stayed with me at the back of the group and told me I wasn't a burden just because I was going slower than the others. Because they were there for me, for the first time in my life, I felt like I could breathe easily in the outdoors.

I'm passionate about fat acceptance and helping others understand that anti-fatness runs rampant in our society so we can start to change things together. The communities that we've built to support and encourage fat people who want to explore the outdoors are entirely opt-in. If you're scared to try hiking, I'm there with you. Alongside us are many more supportive people who understand and will never let you feel like a burden. When I go outdoors, it's to take time to breathe, take notice of how my body is feeling, and to get out of my own head. I want to feel small, in the sense that I'm part of a big, vibrant world pulsating with life—I'm just one small part of it.

KAILA WALTON

(she/her)

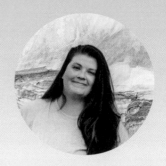

I was very outdoorsy as a kid. I grew up on Denman Island, one of the small Northern Gulf Islands off Vancouver Island in Canada—on the native lands of the Coast Salish, K'omoks, We Wai Kum, We Wai Kai, Homalco, and Tla'amin Nations. As kids we would hang out in the woods a lot, and we spent summers biking to lakes or to friends' houses.

My dad handed down his DSLR camera to me in 2013, which really sparked my interest in photography and hiking. As I got older, I enjoyed the outdoors more. Today, I appreciate it in a different way than I did when I was younger. The beauty and peacefulness of the outdoors is great, as well as the opportunity to photograph wherever I am outside. Being outside helps relieve my stress. I forget about my worries and just focus on what I am doing, whether I'm alone or with some friends. Traveling to cool places I haven't seen before really motivates me to get out—water-falls and sunrises in beautiful places are my favorites—and the hiking itself is a form of joyful movement.

Inclusive and plus-size outdoor community means a great deal to me. I have met some amazing plus-size hikers, photographers, climbers, personal trainers, and other types of athletes through our shared love of the outdoors. One of my most joyous experiences outdoors was in August 2019, when I spent a few days in the Seattle area with a bunch of plus-size friends I'd met on social media. We did various activities outdoors, and I was surrounded the entire time by plus-size or fat women—it changed my life. It's an amazing gift to get to hang out with people who look like you and like to do the things you like to do. This experience really proved to me how much representation matters when it comes to the outdoors (or anything).

Recently, I've gotten into backpacking. It had been on my bucket list for a while, and I figured for my first time, it would feel better to be with a group of experienced plus-size hikers. Though my friends chose a relatively easy trail for my first trip, it turned out to be an unseasonably hot weekend. The conditions were pretty extreme for my first time out, but it did show me what my body was capable of. I'm sure that if the temperatures were more typical for that time of year, we would have been able to finish the hike, but even though we didn't make it all the way to our destination, we found an amazing campground with incredible views. During those two days, the three of us were the largest people on the trail. We got a lot of stares from other people, but for the most part everyone was very friendly.

I wasn't scared before my first backpacking trip, but I was worried that I wouldn't be able to do it. I found it easy to second-guess myself and would think I hadn't trained or prepared myself enough. And maybe I hadn't. But at the same time I told myself, *Your body is capable of a lot of things and lets just see how we do here. We are going to try, and if it doesn't work out, there's always next time.*

As a fat woman, I have found the biggest barrier for all the outdoor activities I'd like to do is access to good technical clothing. I would love to see comfortable hiking pants in bigger plus sizes, good technical tops for layering clothing properly, and nice plus-size puffy jackets. It's really frustrating when there are so few options out there, especially when it comes to backpacking gear. I had such a hard time finding a decent backpacking sleeping bag for myself—one that fit me comfortably and wasn't super heavy—in all my research, I found maybe two brands that each have a single style of plus-size sleeping bag. Finding the right layering clothes for backpacking, which you need when you're out in the mountains, is also seriously hard.

If you want to try backpacking and don't know where to begin, start by looking for gear. If possible, try backpacking for the first time with a friend who has extras you can borrow. The essentials can be expensive,

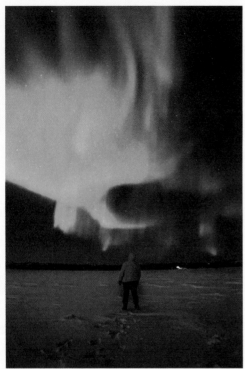

Kaila enjoys photographing herself and others in the outdoors

so build your collection slowly. You'll need a cooking system, backpack, sleeping bag, and sleeping pad. At certain times, you can find those things on sale, which helps a ton.

In addition to a plus-size sleeping bag, you'll need a good sleeping pad in order to be comfortable—look for a nice, lightweight one that is at least two inches thick, maybe more if you can afford it—it will really save your hips. Even better, if you're backpacking in places where you're allowed to use hammocks, I would bring a hammock setup. So comfy! There's lots of information online about hammock backpacking.

Your most vital piece of gear is your backpack. Even though the sales people can be intimidating, make sure you get fitted properly to avoid pain for your shoulders, back, and hips down the line. Hiking poles are amazing. I highly recommend them even just for day hikes. Water is essential for hydration while on any hike, and when you're backpacking, you need to find water wherever you are. I prefer a filtration system to purifying tablets. You won't need as many clothes as you think when backpacking—you're going to smell and be dirty no matter what, so don't waste space and weight on extra clothes.

To physically prepare for backpacking, I like to do a few day hikes with a fairly heavy backpack, or weighted vest. I also do squats when I can to get my body ready.

As physically challenging as backpacking can be, the most challenging experience I've had outdoors is dealing with the pressure of a society that always told me I needed to wait until I was a certain size before I could go backpacking, enjoy day hikes, or do any kind of outdoor activity. I can do all of those things right now! There's no need for me to wait for some future self who is "worthy" enough to do the things I want to do. I am worthy of those things now, and so are you.

I would like to see the general population in the outdoor industry, especially straight-size people, actively speak up and advocate for extended sizing from companies and brands. I also want to see everybody advocating for better plus-size and BIPOC representation in social media campaigns and influencer campaigns. Straight-size people need to amplify the voices of plus-size and marginalized people in the outdoors and talk about how fatphobia and other forms of bigotry harms all people.

Representation is so important. Find a community of people that are similar to you, hang out with them, and ask them for advice or tips. Slowly but surely, plus-size outdoor communities are growing online and creating more in-person meetups. Don't hold yourself back from doing the things you want to do. Don't wait for a future self to enjoy those things. Life is short. Let's do those things now.

CRANESVILLE SWAMP NATURE PRESERVE
TERRA ALTA, WEST VIRGINIA

Erin (she/her)
FGH Chapter: DMV (DC/Maryland/Virginia) region

Cranesville is one of a kind and feels like visiting a completely different part of the country. I highly recommend it for Maryland and West Virginia locals and visitors who want to experience a different kind of forested area. This tranquil preserve is a wonderful place to stop and explore when visiting the nearby Spruce Forest Artisan Village, Deep Creek Lake, Swallow Falls State Park, Coopers Rock State Forest, or any of the beautiful places in the mountains of western Maryland and northeastern West Virginia.

I met Cranesville Swamp for the first time in the winter of 2017. I was staying with a friend at a cabin near Deep Creek Lake, and we decided to explore the nearby Swallow Falls State Park as well as Cranesville Swamp Preserve. I had snow overalls on as we made our way through the heavy drifts, only glimpsing parts of the board-walk beneath our feet. The serene beauty and the complete silence awed me. In

2020, I visited Cranesville again, this time in summer. Wildflowers and marsh plants bloomed and twisted all along the board-walk, and the dirt path was smooth and almost soft beneath me. It felt familiar, especially the tall red pines, which seem to form walls along the trail leading to the boardwalk. In the years between my vis-its, I'd completed a northbound (NOBO), 1,200-mile LASH (Long-Ass Section Hike) on the Appalachian Trail and also embarked on a 10,000-mile solo road trip to explore several national parks. Even

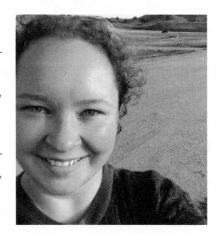

FGH ambassador Erin has hiked all over the country but Cranesville never loses its charm

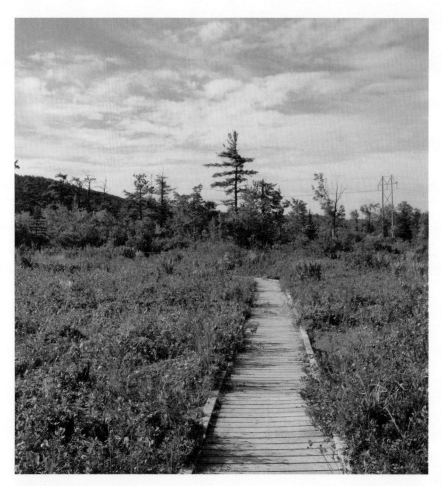

Boardwalk section of the trail

though Cranesville is tiny in comparison, standing on the boardwalk and looking out onto the quiet bog filled me with wonder and left me with a sense of peace.

DISTANCE ROUND TRIP Between 1.2 and 5 miles. There are many interconnected trails, and depending on how much you want to hike, you can explore all of them in one day.

ELEVATION GAIN 36 feet

CELL SERVICE Spotty and unreliable

ADA AND GENERAL ACCESSIBILITY The trails here are not wheelchair accessible. There are no benches, but there are logs comfortable for sitting in some places. This

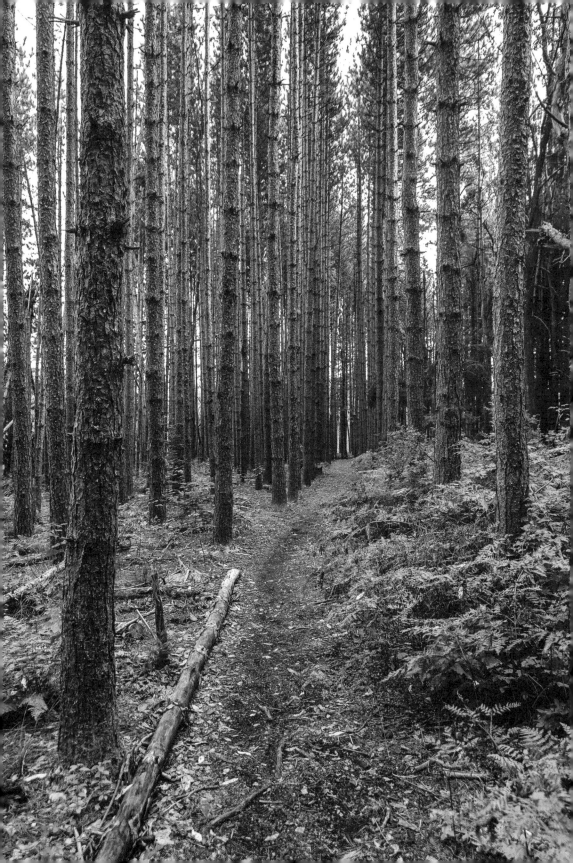

nature preserve is not open to pets. The trails are kid–friendly and manageable for hikers of many skill levels.

BATHROOMS None. There are no bathrooms at this preserve. Plan accordingly and, if you must use the woods as your bathroom, pack it out.

NATIVE LANDS Massawomeck and Osage

TRAIL DESCRIPTION Wildflowers, moss, and marsh plants line the boardwalk, and the tall, elegant trunks of red pine trees line the trails. Many plants that are atypical for this region thrive here because of the unique ecology and geological formation of this place. The dirt trails are mostly smooth and soft with some roots and rocks. The boardwalk is made of hard planks. All the trails can be wet, muddy, or icy, depending on weather conditions.

OFFICIAL PARK ADDRESS Cranesville Swamp Preserve, Terra Alta, WV 26764.

TRAIL NAME Blue Trail and Boardwalk, White Trail

HOW TO FIND THE TRAILHEAD You can find Cranesville Swamp Preserve on any digital map or GPS, and the Nature Conservancy, which manages the preserve, has directions on their website. There is a sign on the road near the entrance. The Blue Trail trailhead starts from the parking lot at the end of Cranesville Road.

ERIN'S HIKING TIP This is a very delicate environment and habitat for many living things—as with all places in nature, please Leave No Trace.

WHEN WE WERE ANIMALS

THAT ESSENTIAL CONNECTION

Humans are animals. We often forget this. We wall ourselves up in boxes—homes, offices, automobiles—and become indoor. Deprived of our instincts to connect with the natural world, we become something other. Our culture presents this indoor life as the only way to live "successfully."

I'm not here to judge or shame anyone for enjoying an indoor life. A life outdoors is not accessible or safe for everyone, and I recognize the privilege I have in living the way I do. My goal is to offer an alternative to the mainstream narrative that we must work, grind, and hustle indoors to be accepted. There are many ways to live a life.

As children, we are told many things. We are told not to get dirty. To be careful. *Don't hurt yourself*, the adults say. We are sheltered behind well-meaning caregivers. We aren't encouraged to be curious. We are taught to behave.

At certain points in my childhood, I was taught manners and etiquette and to sit up straight. But I was also lucky enough to have a mom who would push my siblings and me out the door, telling us to *go play*. I didn't understood then how much of a gift it was to roam the woods without adults, using my imagination and getting lost in worlds I created. Feral cats became my guides through the woods, and I was their queen. Once, an owl swooped down to the low branch of a birch tree and showed me the way to her nest where her babies were small and fuzzy. The train tracks we walked on lead far away from the boring cornfields of my small town.

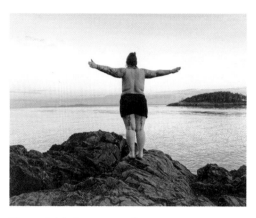
I love to feel the breeze at sunrise

There were a million stories to be told.

As I connect with outdoor spaces as an adult, I remember what it is to be whole. I remember the imaginative play from when I was a child in the woods—an intimate connection to that outdoor space. It can be difficult to maintain that connection now. Yes, we are animals, but we have bills to pay, work to do, and tasks to tidy and maintain our boxes and the people in them. Luckily, we don't need much to be made whole. A yard, a trail, a beach, a wild forest far from any town, or a park in the middle of a city can all provide connection. Why do we humans feel so good after we've spent time outdoors? We are animals and it's in our nature.

Put your bare feet on the sand or grass or wherever you find yourself on the Earth.

Touch the leaves of a tree, trace its lifelines, and note the sensation under your fingers.

Jump into a glacial-fed river on a hot summer day. Yes, it will be cold, but once you're back ashore you'll feel the most alive you've ever felt. Your skin will tingle and you'll feel lit from the inside.

Pick up that rock you just kicked. What is it made of? Taste the place you came from with the tip of your tongue.

Maybe it's raining. Take off your rain jacket. Strip your armor. The armor we are told we should always keep on—remove it. Feel the cool drops on your warm mammal skin.

Close your eyes and feel the warm sun on your face. You can do this anywhere—city, town, or wild space.

Take note of what you see. What you emote. What you awaken within yourself once you've made an intentional connection to the natural world. Your senses are now wide open. You are alive. A remarkable thing.

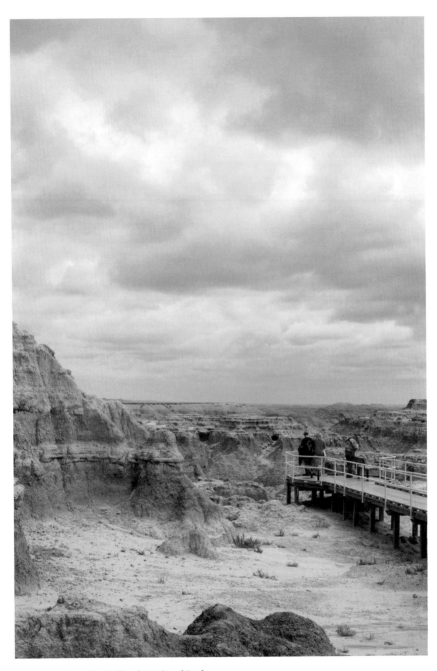

A boardwalk trail in Badlands National Park

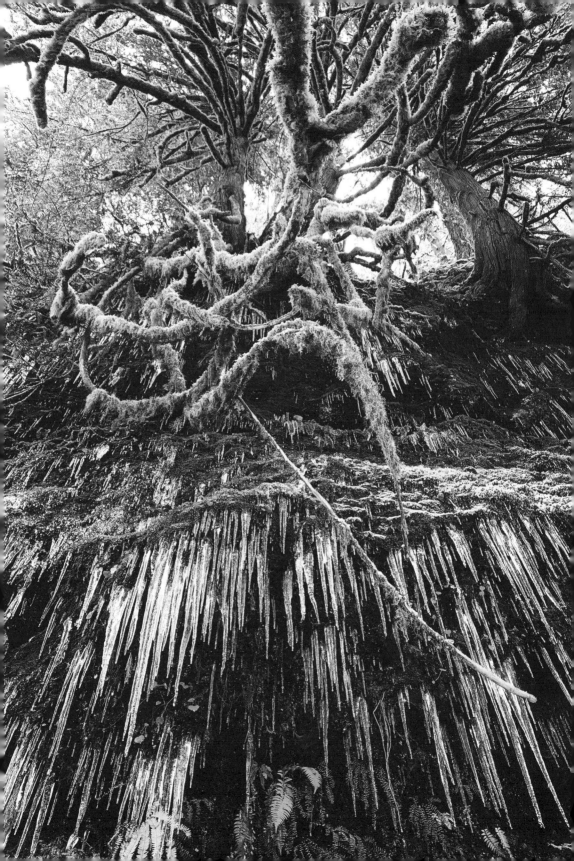

We humans feel the effects of modern life on our mental and emotional well-being. We are stressed and anxious. When we lack a connection to nature, fear and anger are always near the surface, but when we are outdoors, the chemicals in our brains behave differently. By honoring the land and our connections to it, our emotions, thoughts, and habits become nourishing rather than harmful. Our instincts aren't only to survive but also to feed the curious, mammal child within us.

At this point in my life, I am outside most of the day, every day. My life is no longer walled up in a box. When I gave up the safety and comfort of an apartment for a van, I gave myself the gift of realizing:

I am an animal that needs to place my bare feet on wet grass, even if that means I step on a few jagged rocks.

I am an animal that craves knowing the names for trees, plants, flowers, birds, and other mammals. It seems a human thing to crave, but curiosity and knowledge benefit us.

I seek to remember the patterns and migrations of life changes as they were before modern ways of being stripped me of what I must have once known. The energy I absorb outdoors has been instrumental in improving my quality of life. Joy is easier for me to cultivate under the watchful eyes of a hawk that soars above trees older than I am. This outdoor life is not always easy, nor does everybody understand it, but it is a good life as a curious human animal open to the possibilities of every single day.

CELESTE MICK

(she/her)

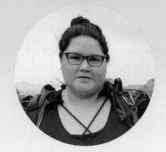

I wasn't really outdoorsy growing up. I only did a hike and went camping once as a kid—it was a nice experience, but I was more into swimming and never felt the need to be in nature much. It wasn't until I found myself emotionally lost and broken that I had an urge to explore and get lost in nature—that's when nature healed me.

When I started hiking in 2013, I didn't have any knowledge of what gear I needed or really anything related to hiking. I just felt compelled to reconnect with myself during a difficult time in my life. I was feeling pretty lost and unhappy in my own skin, and I thought hiking would make me feel empowered and alive again. My perception of nature changed through the experiences I had outdoors. Today, the energy that nature brings to my body and soul inspires me to get outdoors often. It's happened so many times—I might be in a bad mood at the beginning of a hike, but I always return to the trailhead bright as the California sunshine.

Although most of my outdoor experiences have been extremely positive, there have been times in which I've been approached by people who tell me that it's good I'm hiking to lose weight, or who have felt the need to provide unsolicited advice about how I could lose weight while I'm out on a trail. I've had people say I shouldn't be hiking this or that mountain and make inappropriate comments about my body. These comments create a barrier for me when I want to go hiking. I shouldn't have to face this type of discrimination when all I want is to hike the same trails as everyone else. Nature welcomes us all, but our society has created an exclusive environment where many of us don't feel welcome.

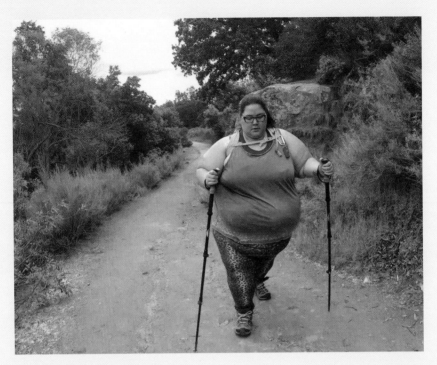

Celeste hikes to connect with herself

When I first started hiking, I didn't see any fat representation in outdoor media at all. The situation has improved over the years, but we still have a long way to go. It is vital that outdoor brands expand to sizes beyond 3XL. Outdoorsy people like me, who wear sizes bigger than 3X feel excluded. We want to be able to find clothes and gear that will let us enjoy the outdoors in the bodies we're are in right now. We shouldn't have to "earn" good gear by losing weight.

To me a brand that expands their sizes but doesn't feature people who represent that extended range in their advertising is not worth my investment. I used to be afraid to go to outdoor gear stores because I wasn't represented anywhere in any of their ads—no plus-size people were. I want to see outdoor stores be much more inclusive in their marketing. Most of the major companies in this market have the resources to create seminars, forums, and classes where people can learn about inclusion, race issues in the outdoors, and acceptance. If they wanted to, they could put more

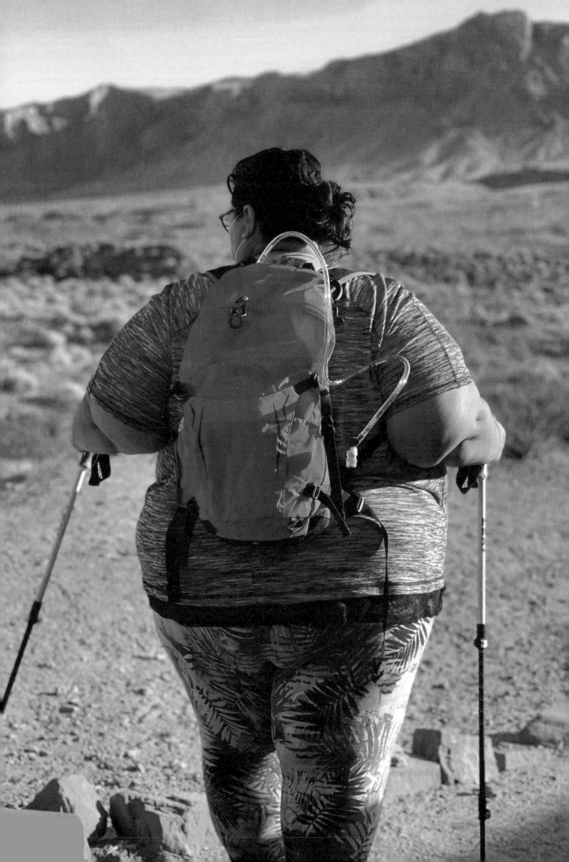

of an emphasis on education about social issues and how marginalized people are affected by not being represented in the outdoors. Inclusive outdoor communities like Fat Girls Hiking are a strong foundation for anyone who doesn't feel seen or represented by the big outdoor brands.

My first hike was the most joyous outdoor experience I've ever had. I was so unprepared! I made it to the top, what I thought of as the end, and enjoyed the sunset. Then it got dark. I was trapped on the mountain. I was so scared and thought about stopping and just sleeping in the open, but I kept going back to the trailhead. Hours later, I saw a reflection—it was my car window. When I got home, all dirty, tired, and sore, I felt so strong—I was always told that this hike would be too hard for me (And it was hard!), but I did it.

It's completely okay to feel intimidated, scared, or afraid when hiking for the first time. Remember to take it one step at a time. Take it slow—it's not about how much time or distance you put in. Outdoor recreation is about how you feel once you're in it. On that first hike, I thought that driving to the parking lot in my car was brave enough—when I came back from the trail in the dark, I realized this was a new me.

PAPAGO BUTTES
PHOENIX, ARIZONA

Amy Rios-Richardson (she/her)
FGH chapter: Phoenix, Arizona

I'm grateful for the opportunities I've had in the last several years to get to know my body through being in nature. I claim my space in the world! I love clumsily navigating my way through beginner trails and getting to know how my body moves, heals, and grows stronger.

Double Butte Trail is one of the first hikes my wife and I tried out when we moved to Phoenix. It is so accessible, right in the midst of the city, with ample parking, and makes a perfect quick escape from the nine-to-five hustle. You can see the park's red sandstone buttes sticking up out of the desert landscape from just about any highway in Phoenix, so to be standing between them is a wonderful feeling of connection.

The FGH Phoenix chapter did our inaugural hike here, and we had a blast taking photos in front of the buttes and getting to know each other. This hike will always hold a special place in my heart, because it's where I found my FGH community. Though I usually visit late in the morning or early in the evening so I haven't seen it myself, I've heard that watching the sunrise and the sunset here is stunning.

This trail is perfect for beginner hikers and experienced hikers alike. For beginners, you're not too far from civilization in case you get nervous and want to turn back. For more experienced hikers, you can easily veer off the trail and explore the buttes' nooks and crannies.

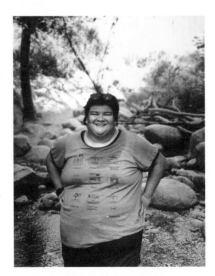

In addition to hiking, Amy enjoys kayaking, camping, swimming, and snorkeling

DISTANCE ROUND TRIP 2.3 miles

ELEVATION GAIN 50 feet

CELL SERVICE Yes

ADA AND GENERAL ACCESSIBILITY The trail is partially paved, but mostly dirt and somewhat rocky—it may be accessible for some types of wheelchairs, mobility devices, and walkers. The grade is never more than 5 percent.

BATHROOMS None

NATIVE LANDS Akimel O'odham, Hohokam, and O'odham Jeweḍ

TRAIL DESCRIPTION One minute you're driving through the bustling city of Phoenix, the next you're in the midst of beautiful red sandstone formations. This hike's main features are these stunning buttes that pop out of the desert. Look up and you'll see folks who have climbed the buttes trying to capture perfect photos of the sunset or sunrise. Depending on the season, you may also see wildflowers. Hikers, trail runners, and bikers all use this trail.

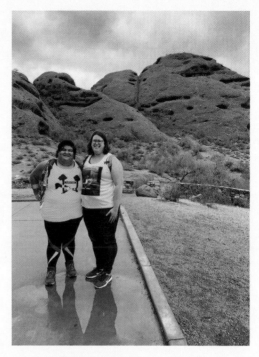

Amy on the trail with her wife

OFFICIAL PARK ADDRESS Papago West Park, West Buttes Parking Lot, 626 North Gavin Parkway, Phoenix AZ 85008

TRAIL NAME Double Butte Trail

HOW TO FIND THE TRAILHEAD The trail starts at the north end of the West Buttes Parking Lot off Papago Park Road.

AMY'S HIKING TIPS Enjoy the picnic tables at the beginning and middle of this trail—pack a snack, a lunch, or just take a breather. There's a water fountain at the picnic tables.

JOLIE VARELLA

(she/her)

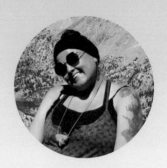

I am a citizen of the Tule River Yokut and Paiute Nations. I come from Payahuunadü, the place of flowing water. I am an Indigenous activist, and I care very deeply for my people and the land we belong to.

When we were kids, my cousins and I would ride our bikes with our inner tubes to go to our swimming spot, properly named the Indian Hole. We'd swim in the creeks and float down to the elders building. I was probably eleven years old when I would load up my fishing pole, crickets, and radio and hop two barbed wire fences to get to my fishing spot. I'd sit for hours by myself, then bring home a stringer of fish for my mom and dad who love to eat pugwi.

In my mid to late twenties, I was going through a hard time with depression, bipolar disorder, and anxiety. I would get up early and go hiking by myself—I found that while on my own outdoors, I could be open with myself and think about abandonment trauma from my childhood. I would have the most amazing experiences hiking up steep elevations in beautiful surroundings, and I always felt so good afterward. Hiking became a way to improve my mental health. It also opened me up to trying other things on my own. I began adding to the list of things I could do alone: first hiking then eating out then going to the movies.

For ten years I was a waitress, but since founding Indigenous Women Hike in 2017, I have been able to make community organizing my fulltime heart's work. I lead group hikes. I also sit on two boards of directors and do speaking engagements and panels. I started Indigenous Women Hike with a vision to hike the Nüümü Poyo, or "People's Trail" (which most people today call the John Muir Trail), as part of a great healing journey and ceremony. Our mission has expanded to include raising awareness of Indigenous issues and educating people about the history of the lands on which they recreate—namely how my people and other Native Nations were violently removed to create "wilderness" places.

I never saw myself as an outdoorsy person. Not in the way that you see portrayed by the outdoor industry. But thinking about the ways I interacted with the land growing up makes me smile and feel grateful. What makes going on a hike in a National Park more outdoorsy than being out on the land gathering traditional foods? And how is a walk in a city park any less outdoorsy than a walk in a National Park? It's all sacred land.

I remember once while I was hiking, I went off the path to rest and found grinding stones. Whenever I'm outdoors, I know that the trees remember who I am. *You have your great great grandmothers eyes*, they'll say. When I'm on the trail, I'm growing that connection to my ancestors. There can often be a lack of consent with taking from the land. The ancestors remind me to give back to the land, that our connection to the land needs to be a reciprocal relationship.

The brutal history and genocide that happened on the land can combine with the mainstream culture of outdoor recreation to make me feel like I don't actually belong outside. Eurocentric values that stem from colonization and removal of Indigenous people created a narrative that my body doesn't belong not only because it is Indigenous but also because it is fat and therefore doesn't adhere to Eurocentric beauty values. Actually, bodies of any size belong on the land. I'm usually the fattest person on any given trail. Even though I don't look like your "typical" hiker—or at least what people think of when they think of a hiker, thanks to a lack of representation in the outdoor industry—I have a huge sense of pride when I'm hiking. I say to myself, *my fat body is up here*. I did this.

Some might look at me and judge my body, but the thing that hurts the most is when they refuse to acknowledge that my people were displaced from their homelands. This denial, preferring to almost pretend that Indigenous people don't exist, is harmful to my well-being and that of my people. Failing to acknowledge Indigenous history and refusing to

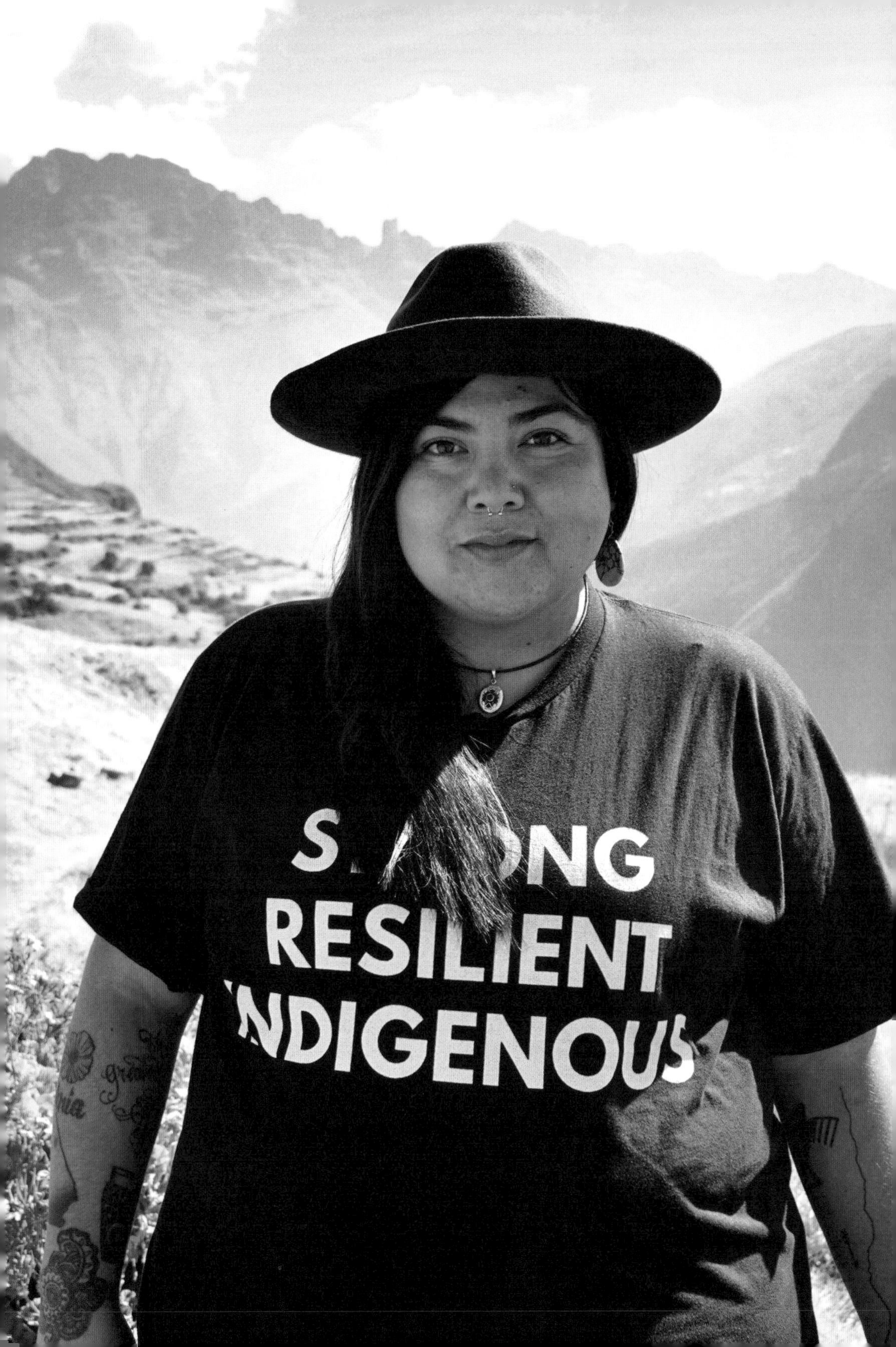
RESILIENT

acknowledge us as the original stewards of the land is hurtful. I can feel the barrier, but it does not hold me back, because I know my ancestors were out on this land.

Hiking saved my life. Hiking is what I needed to do to get through my life. Things got even better as I learned more about Indigenous history on the trail. Getting outdoors is an act of love—it reconnects me with myself and builds and nourishes my inherent connection to the land. When I'm out on the trail, I remember everything the land does for every aspect of our lives.

I want to pass all that I have learned and experienced to younger generations. I want to let young Indigenous kids know we have always stewarded the land and tell them to be proud of the land they come from. I didn't have a good idea of what being Indigenous meant as a kid, and I hope to change that for the next generation. Our wellness kids camps aim to inspire exploration of what being Indigenous means.

I have also created and continue to maintain a free, outdoor-gear library for people in my community. I remember when I got my first hiking pack—I felt like I fit in more on the trails. I know "fitting in" isn't the priority when it comes to gear, but having the right tools does affect our ability to feel comfortable. Everybody deserves access to the things that make us safe, physically and mentally, on the trail. The gear library is a way to break down one of the barriers my community faces when accessing outdoor recreation. I've seen families go on their first camping trip using gear from the library. That's an experience they wouldn't have been able to share otherwise.

The land does not discriminate. All bodies belong. It's up to us to create a healthy and reciprocal relationship with it. Indigenous bodies belong on the land. Get out on it when you can—we all deserve to get the good medicine the land offers.

ANNETTE RICHMOND

(she/her)

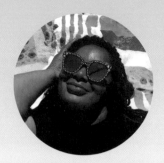

My most joyous and most challenging experience outdoors, both physically and emotionally, was hiking from Little Petra to the Monastery in Jordan. I've always felt like if things got too difficult on a hike, I could turn around and go back the way I came. But on a long desert hike, no matter where you turn, there is only more desert. I was traveling with a group of new friends and was nervous I would hold everyone back. The hike was nearly five hours through the desert in the sun. I shared my concerns with the tour guide and the people who ran the trip, and, in the end, I did the hike with their reassurances. We got through it together, and

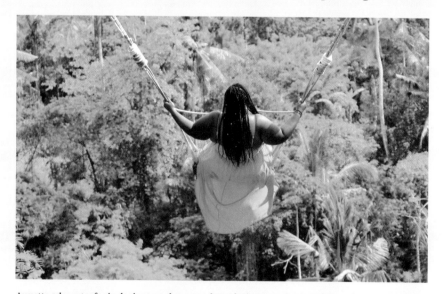

Annette advocates for inclusive travel spaces—here she is on a swing in Bali

I wasn't the last person! I felt invigorated afterward and so proud of myself but not without a few tears and conquered fears.

As a kid, I went to camp every summer, which I think makes me outdoorsy by default. I hiked, camped, and rode horses. I didn't always love it while I was doing it, though. I remember one summer I didn't go to camp, I went to Arizona with my god mom and stayed on her mother's farm. Every morning, I would get the eggs from the chicken coop and feed the pigs, horses, and donkeys. That summer was the first time I got bucked off a horse. I also built a legit outdoor fort that was like a mansion. It took all day and just as we were getting settled in our sleeping

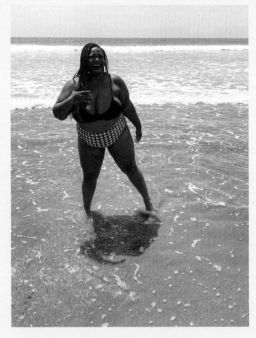

Annette founded a fat-positive summer camp for adults to help create uplifting, empowering memories

bags, ready to sleep in the fort we'd built, we saw a scorpion. We ran inside so fast! By the end of summer, being out in nature always created the best memories.

As a Black person, I oftentimes don't feel safe in the outdoors. I was recently driving through Big Sur on a road trip to Los Angeles, and I had so much anxiety about driving through a state park at night. I decided to make as few stops as possible and to keep an eye on my gas tank. I don't feel safe alone in the woods at night, especially because cell phone reception is often poor in these areas. Wondering how I might possibly contact someone if I encounter an emergency is terrifying to me. So many tragedies have only been acknowledged after they've been shared live on social media.

Still, I love hiking in Northern California. The redwoods, crisp air, and views are stunning. Because it's where I grew up, it feels so familiar to me and like it's the epitome of the great outdoors. I try to spend a few hours a

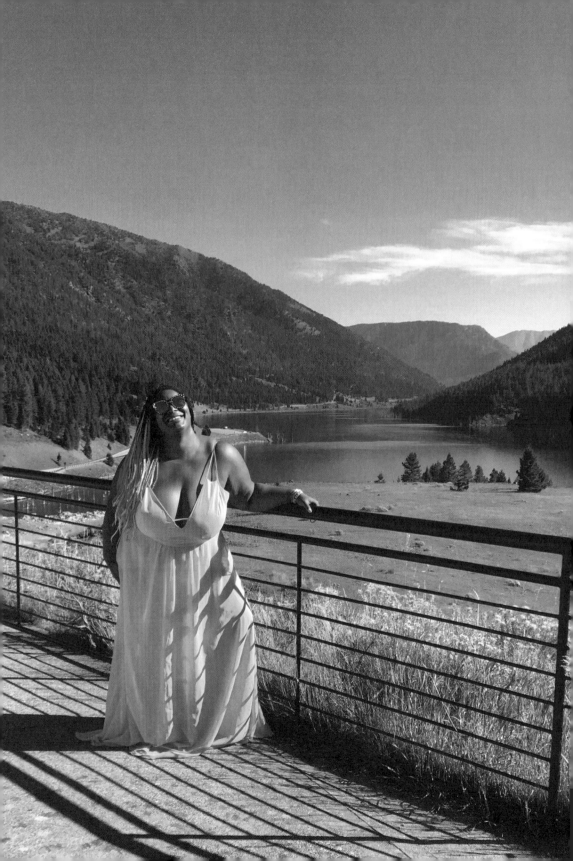

week outdoors—I go to the beach to sunbathe, meditate, and swim, and I go for walks regularly.

When it's time to purchase a kayak, tent, sleeping bag, sleeping pad, chair, or weatherproof items that fit me, I must become a detective. Which is frustrating because fat people like me are active. Don't limit us—we're limitless! The industry really needs to make all types of outdoor gear for bigger people, including climbing harnesses, kayaks, zip lines, and any other fun outdoor activity that people in smaller bodies don't even have to think twice about in terms of accessibility. In addition to the sizing of gear, there is still a lot of work to be done when it comes to making the outdoors accessible to people with disabilities. A general lack of representation for marginalized people in outdoor spaces, including among park rangers and tour guides, perpetuates ideas about who "belongs" there. The goal should be diversity not only among visitors but among those who represent parks and natural spaces as well.

I get myself outside mainly to relax. Being in nature helps me feel grounded—even though I sweat *a lot*, and mosquitoes are obsessed with me. Sometimes, it's not always the most pleasant, but I continue to do it anyway because the positive experiences outweigh the negative ones. I know that simply getting outside daily, smelling the fresh air, and feeling the breeze on my skin helps my mental, emotional, and physical health. It's one of the easiest ways I can take care of myself.

POINT MUGU STATE PARK
MALIBU, CALIFORNIA

Kelly Estabrook (she/her)
FGH chapter: Los Angeles, California

When I was a kid, I would ride my bike around the neighborhood and tell stories to the trees. I love the magic of nature. I love how hiking and being in nature can bring you very deep into the present moment. When I'm among trees, all my worries melt away.

Hiking is therapeutic and makes me so happy. I think it's fascinating what our bodies can do and where they can take us. I enjoy learning something new about myself or the world every time I go on a hike.

The Scenic and Overlook Trails Loop is my favorite in Point Mugu State Park. The first time I hiked this trail was to celebrate my birthday with my mom, sister, and son. We had a great time and loved the views. This is definitely a family-friendly trail.

DISTANCE ROUND TRIP 2.7 miles

ELEVATION GAIN 425 feet

CELL SERVICE Yes

ADA AND GENERAL ACCESSIBILITY This is not an ADA-accessible hike. There are no benches or places to rest along the trail.

BATHROOMS Yes. There are gendered bathrooms at the trailhead.

NATIVE LANDS Chumash and Ventureño

TRAIL DESCRIPTION Along the trail to the ridge, you will see the rolling Malibu hills, part of the Santa Monica Mountains. Reaching the ridge reveals a beautiful vista of the Pacific Ocean.

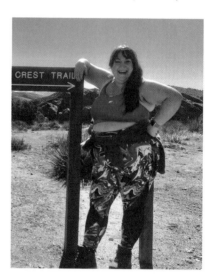

Kelly likes to hike with her mom, sister, and son

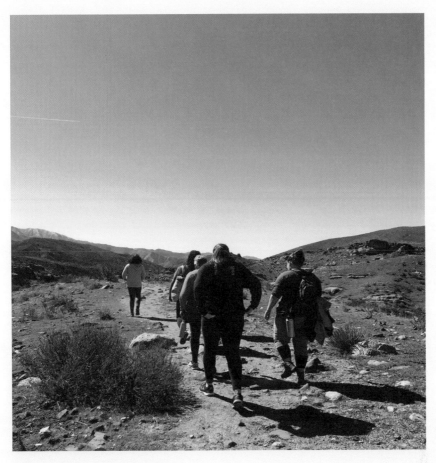

FGH LA enjoy the view from the trail

OFFICIAL PARK ADDRESS Point Mugu's official address is on the Pacific Coast High-way, but the Scenic and Overlook Trails start at Sycamore Canyon Campground, Malibu, CA 90265

TRAIL NAME Scenic and Overlook Trails

HOW TO FIND THE TRAILHEAD Park in the day use area for the Sycamore Canyon Campground on the north side of the Pacific Coast Highway for $10 or along the PCH for free if you find a spot near the entrance. Walk north along the paved road through the campground until you get to the dirt Sycamore Canyon Fire Road. From there, follow the signs to Scenic Trail.

CHANGE ALWAYS COMES

—

THE RESTLESSNESS INSIDE

wake before dawn and drive to a cliffside viewpoint to watch the sunrise over the ocean. The colors of the world around me change subtly. Time moves on through watercolor skies. From black to navy to dark purple to a pink-peach-orange then a white-yellow mixed with blue. It's all mixed with blue. The blue of the sky. The blue of the ocean. The blue in my eyes that sees the vast endlessness of it all. As the sun breaks past the horizon, there's a relief and also sadness. I want day to come, but I want a slow-motion transition. The shifting colors smooth the butterflies in my gut. The scenery change plays like a happy montage. A comedy before tragic reality sets in? No. That anxiety is cured with the sun, the moon, the tide, the colors.

We moved around a lot when I was a kid. I packed my Alyssa Milano posters and push-button typewriter and got used to laying new roots and making new friends. How, as an adult, am I supposed to want to stay in the permanent box of an apartment or house?

When I lived in a city, I found it hard to calm the need for change that often overwhelmed me. Sometimes I'd dye my hair. Sometimes I'd take a midnight drive down to the Columbia River. Sometimes I'd rearrange my apartment.

Maybe I crave more than what's in front of me right now. Maybe I have to feed an innate longing for growth inside myself. Or maybe my urge to change can never be sated because of how I grew up. What is this

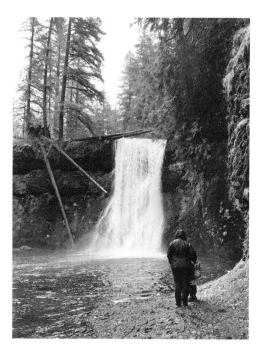

Instill a love of nature in future generations by sharing magical spots, like this one at Silver Falls State Park

internal creature that thrashes to be fed? Why do I have to dive head first into every wave?

When I'm in the forest, there are hidden love notes under every leaf. Entire libraries are bound in the bark of several-hundred-year-old trees. Under the forest canopy, the humid microclimate drips on my skin, tired with urban silt. With stubborn fortitude, I keep movement in my feet and run my fingers along the moss on the tree bark, still wet from yesterday's rain.

The constant shifting of the outdoors calms me. Everything is different seasonally. If I can stay in one place long enough, I can watch the change happen.

A forest understory covered in yellow big-leaf-maple confetti. Those leaves, bigger than my head, drip with fresh rain. My first fall in Portland, over a decade ago, I saw those leaves and was mesmerized by their size. I had never seen leaves that big in my life. How are they real?

I think about my seasonal routines.

In fall, I visit the famous Japanese maple in the Portland Japanese Garden. Photographers from around the world visit it too, mesmerized by its orange and red leaves—lens flares splash artistically across its wiry branches. I go to the Hoyt Arboretum visitor center and ask which trails have colorful leaves. I find the maples and spend an afternoon among them.

In winter, the mud cakes thick on my hiking boots. I once hated, really hated, having mud or dirt on me. There was a whole phase in my late twenties and early thirties in which I just could not deal with bugs or dirt

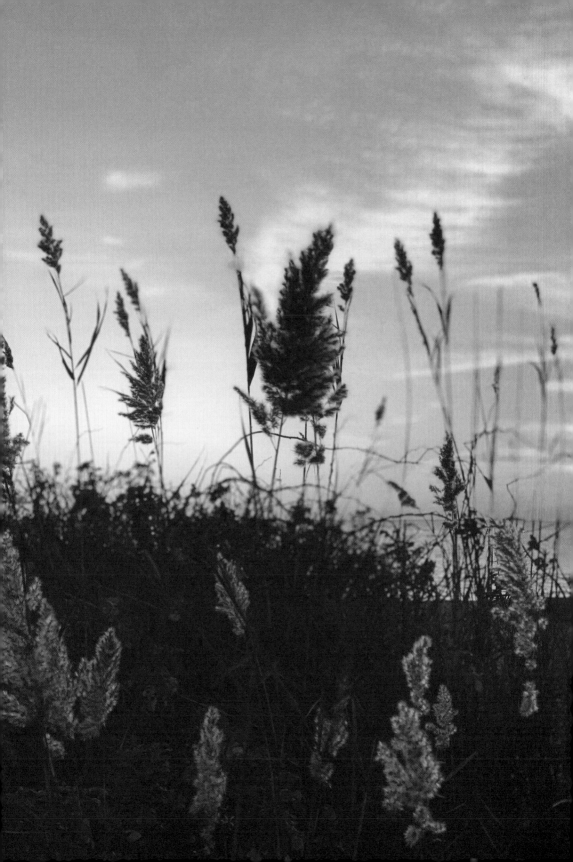

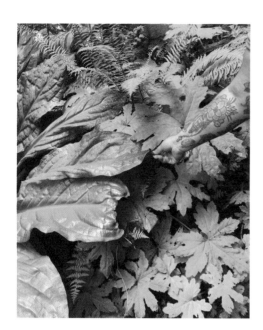

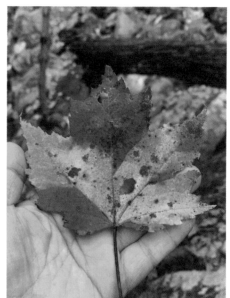

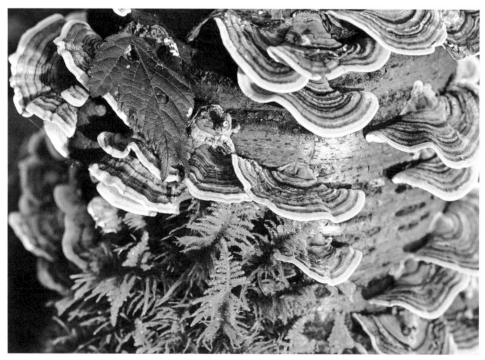

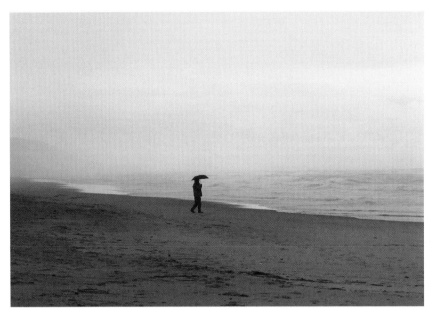

On the Oregon coast, beach umbrellas mean something a little different

or sand. Anything that made me feel uncomfortable or put out in any way I would not try again. Sand in my bathing suit? Nope!

Now, I see mud on my boots as a sign of a day that's been lived—it means I've gotten into the muck of the world and likely smiled at life's unpredictability. I have to remind myself to clean my feet before I go to sleep so I don't get sand in my bed. Mossy branches lining trails, blown down by winter winds, are treasures I use to decorate my dashboard. I embrace the rain.

In spring, trillium greets her friends along the trail—balsamroot, purple lupine, foxglove, and those tiny sweet orange Columbia tiger lilies. I travel with a rain jacket at all times in spring. You just never know. The rain comes swift. A pleasant sunny day can turn into a downpour or that ever-so-charming mist that just makes everything wet. If you've visited the Pacific Northwest, you know what I mean. We have many types of rain here. The big plop drops that seem to miss every step you take. The dreary gray. The it-has-rained-for-twenty-five-consecutive-days conversations

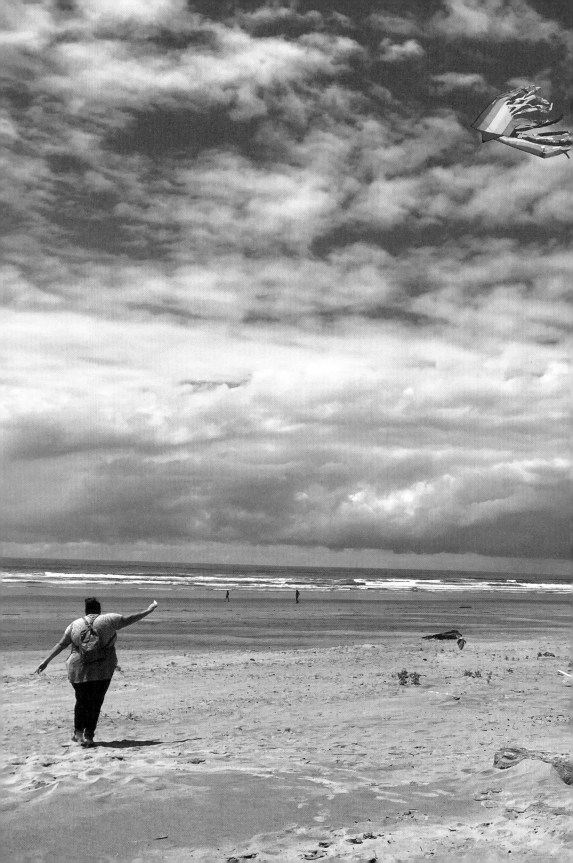

that punctuate every interaction—with gas station attendants, therapists, best friends meeting up for a late afternoon movie.

In summer, my beloved moss dries and changes colors. The morning fog burns off, and by noon the sky is bright blue—sky blue. The beaches become lined with tourists who think, *Maybe I should move here. It's so nice here, it's cheap and people are friendly.* People who visit Oregon in summer are charmed. Why wouldn't they be? It's a magical place. I spend the entire summer barefooted or in flip-flops. I take dips in nearby rivers in the late afternoon. I watch the sunset over the ocean every night. But the real lure for me, being the rebellious little shit that

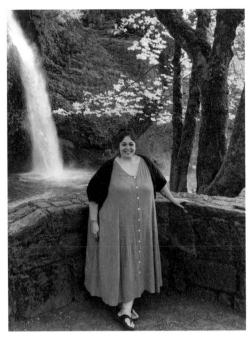

Ginamarie near Horsetail Falls, which is right beside the Historic Columbia River Highway

I am, is the rainy winter months when you can go an entire day without seeing another human. The empty beaches are a gift, ok? And, the loneliness can be so real. I love it.

Each season has a home inside me. Each season pulls me outdoors to experience the change that happens before my eyes, to comfort that inner child who just wants to be still awhile. That child who can never be still. I no longer think of the constant need for change as a bad thing. It's just a thing that makes me who I am. Once I embraced the outdoors, my arms were open to the change that occurs around me everywhere, every day, every second, if only I open my eyes and my heart to its gifts.

OSWALD WEST STATE PARK
OREGON COAST

Ellen (she/her)
FGH Chapter: Portland, Oregon

I love hiking, backpacking, painting, gardening, reading, anything outside. I just love being outside—it's how I reset and connect with myself. My favorite thing about nature is the light and how it changes depending on the time of day or weather. It's the perfect reminder of natural cycles and that shifts are a normal part of life.

What I love about the trails at Oswald West State Park is that they're go-with-the-flow trails. You can show up to the park without an agenda and be in the moment. It's also one of the few areas on the Oregon coast that isn't developed.

DISTANCE ROUND TRIP Short Sands Beach hike is 1.2 miles. The hike to Kramer Memorial picnic area (an overlook of Short Sands beach) is 1 mile. The Cape Falcon hike is 5 miles.

ELEVATION GAIN 100 feet for Short Sands Beach; 300 feet for Cape Falcon; minimal elevation on the hike to Kramer Memorial

CELL SERVICE No

ADA AND GENERAL ACCESSIBILITY Cape Falcon is the main trail from the largest of the parking lots to the picnic area called Kramer Memorial—it is paved and packed down, with a couple dips in the pavement that may be tricky, but it's a relatively well-maintained trail. It has downed logs to sit on and a picnic area with several tables and benches. The hikes that continue on to Cape Falcon and Devil's Cauldron are not ADA accessible, and there are no places available to rest along the

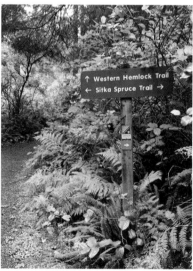

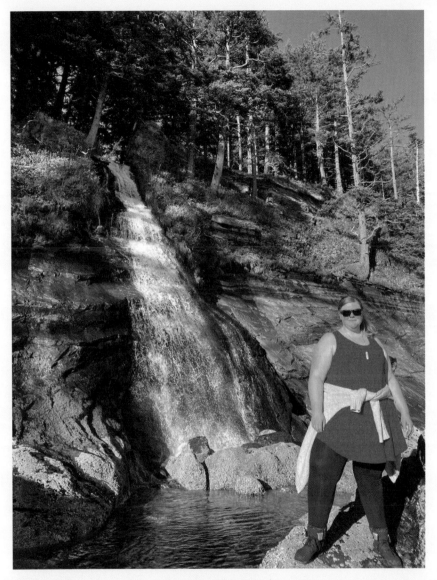

FGH Minnesota ambassador Ani at Blumenthal Falls, which flows right onto Short Sands Beach

way. The trail to Short Sands Beach is not ADA accessible but does have both picnic tables and benches at the end of the trail with a view of the ocean.

BATHROOMS Yes. In the North Short Sands Beach parking area (the largest parking lot on the eastside of Highway 101) there is a gendered, ADA–accessible bathroom.

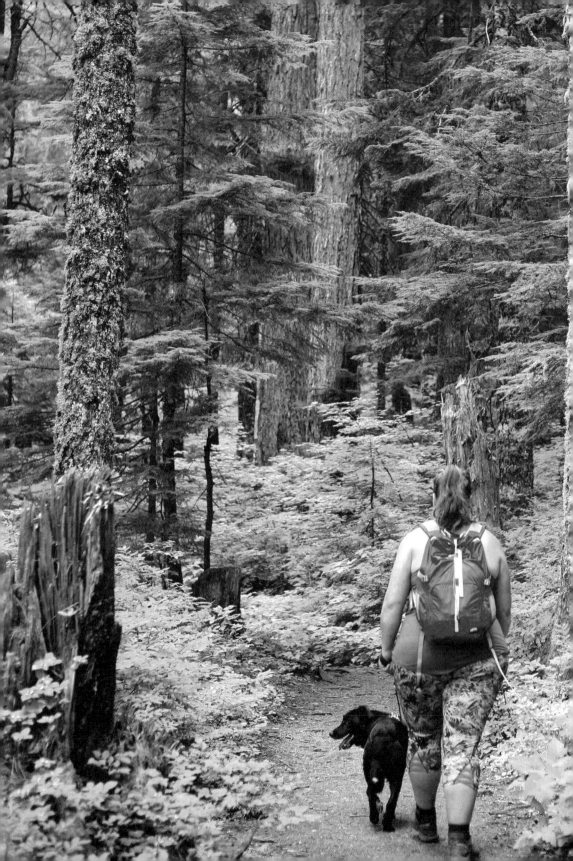

There is also a gendered bathroom at the ocean viewpoint near Short Sands Beach—it is not ADA accessible and the stalls are small.

NATIVE LANDS Nehalem and the Confederated Tribes of Grand Ronde

TRAIL DESCRIPTION The Short Sands hike was once a walk-in campground and is now a maze of short trails that lead you to the ocean. The hike is framed by two creeks, which amble through an old-growth rainforest to a beach sandwiched between bluffs. Short Sands is a surfing beach, and you're likely to see surfers jogging down the trail to warm up before hitting the water—they'll call out to tell you if they're coming up on your right or left as they pass you. If you want to head up the bluffs, you can take in views of Cape Falcon or the Devil's Cauldron by picking up trails on both the north and south ends of the beach. From the main parking area you can take a paved and packed-down ADA-friendly trail to a picnic area with a view of the ocean. The beach-access trail is built from rocks and old railroad ties in loose sand. The main parking area has free brochures with a map of all the hike options.

OFFICIAL PARK ADDRESS Oswald West State Park, Highway 101, Arch Cape, OR 97102

TRAIL NAME South Beach Access Trail and Cape Falcon Trail

HOW TO FIND THE TRAILHEAD The park has three parking lots: Cape Falcon Trailhead parking lot, North Short Sands Trailhead parking lot (the largest lot, on the east side of Highway 101), and South Short Sands Trailhead parking lot. Parking is not allowed on highway shoulders. Please note that this area can be busy, especially on weekends and during summer.

ELLEN'S HIKING TIPS Pack a picnic and enjoy the ocean views for a while. If you take the trails to the beach, walk north to Blumenthal Falls, at the far north end of the beach and reachable at low tide. Check the rocky tide pools for sea urchins and anemones.

KAILEY KORNHAUSER

(she/her)

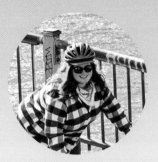

As a midwestern kid, I was fortunate to grow up with a dad who prioritized camping and romanticized the American West. Our primary form of outdoor recreation was RV travel to midwestern lakes and National Parks. I interacted with the outdoors as a sightseer—in many ways that is still how I interact with it, but I traded the RV for a bike. I biked as a kid in the neighborhood and picked it back up as a college student who couldn't afford a car. Slowly, I transitioned from a reluctant bike commuter to an avid bikepacker. Outside of seeing the world through bicycle travel, my other passions in life are environmental policy and working with communities to build capacity to adapt to the impacts of climate change.

When I first started bikepacking, the cost of a bike and all the expensive camping gear that goes along with it was a huge barrier. Another was figuring out which clothes would work for me. I wear padded shorts for comfort, and it took a few tries to find the right size and feel. Then there are the cultural barriers; I think those are the hardest to overcome. For a long time I never saw anyone in a larger body riding a bike—in the media or out in the world—and it felt like that meant people like me didn't ride bikes. Because I live in a fairly small and homogenous town, I ended up finding most of my outdoor community online. It seems counterintuitive to search the web for outdoor friends, but for me it's a way to find folks who look like me and share the same struggles and joys in biking. Many of my newfound friends ride bikes as a way to make progressive change in their wider communities and approach the outdoors in a healing and joyful way. I take this community spirit with me mentally every time I bike and I feel those friends with me when I'm having hard moments or celebrating success.

Bikepacking can be both joyful and extremely challenging. I love how far I can travel on a bike and how long it takes me to go that distance. I find that my favorite natural places change in each phase of my life based on the communities I'm working with (right now, I'm loving the Oregon Coast Range). I find joy in the physical feeling of moving my bike, and the surprise of how far my body can take me. There are amazing moments—sailing down a mountain pass or pedaling through a canyon. And there are hard moments—pushing my bike up a hill or saddle sores after nine-plus hours of riding.

I sometimes receive judgmental comments masked as compliments. People will say things like *You got this!* to me as they ride past but say nothing to my friends in smaller bodies. A lot of other bikers assume I'm a beginner or congratulate me for *getting out there*. These remarks assume that I bike as a way to lose weight, or that I lack the expertise of a person in a smaller body. The outdoors is not inherently exclusive, but the

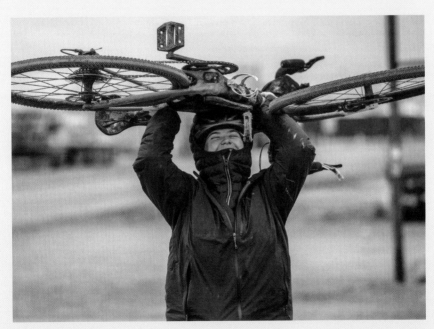

Kailey knows her body's strength

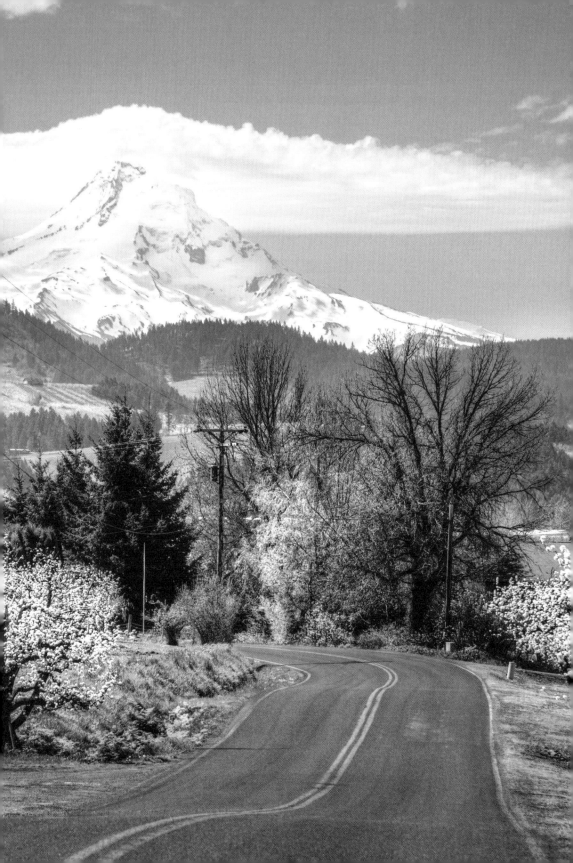

culture surrounding it is—behaviors and attitudes tied to outdoor recreation haven't always been welcoming of diverse groups of people, and the traditional Western approach to outdoor spaces is one that's white, masculine, straight, and thin.

That being said, the outdoors is for everyone, and if you find that you don't see anyone who looks like you on your hike/bike/surf/float/etc., try looking for that community online. When I started biking and didn't see anyone who looked like me, I felt an oppressive need to prove to everyone around me, and myself, that I was a "real" biker. The thing is, if you are a person on a bike, no matter what type of bike, then you are a biker. Outdoor recreation is just supposed to be a fun time outside, to do what feels good with people who make you feel good doing it. Also, yes, the bike saddle will hurt your butt—there are ways around it, but the unfortunate secret is that your butt will always hurt a little bit.

I bike most often as a form of transportation, as a way to get outside after work or to pick up a cinnamon roll from the local bakery. My bike also connects me to natural places. I bikepack as a way to show myself what I'm capable of, and to see remote parts of the world slowly. It's this perfect balance of moving slowly across great distances that keeps me coming back. My most joyous outdoor experience, overall, is looking back at all the amazing places my bike has taken me and all the wonderful people with whom I've had the pleasure of pedaling along the way.

GINAMARIE

(she/her)

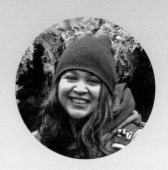

Growing up, my family did a ton of camping. I was taught to respect nature and revel in all its gifts. I loved to hike and explore my surroundings while collecting fallen treasures. As far back as I can remember, I've preferred to be outdoors and now, amid my busy daily life, I still try to get outdoors every day.

My passion in life is to help give a voice to marginalized people. Especially the younger generations, as they are often dismissed. I am an advocate for disabled people, LGBTQ+ people, and BIPOC. My work centers around the personal care and well-being of disabled people.

My favorite place in nature is anywhere I can wrap my arms around a big ol' tree and smell the moss. When I connect with nature, it calms the stresses of daily life. It's a place to meditate and ground myself to gain perspective and focus. I also just love being surrounded by nature's gifts. The Oregon coast is another of my favorite places. The air, the sun, the wind, the rain, the wildlife, and the foliage all inspire me to get outdoors.

I have experienced bigotry related to my size and race in my daily life, which has prevented me from putting myself out where I could be ridiculed for taking up space. Thankfully, there are groups for fat and marginalized folks to reclaim their presence outdoors.

The outdoors in its natural state is welcoming to all, however, I absolutely do not feel represented in mainstream outdoor media or within the outdoor industry. The industry could be welcoming by carrying clothing and safety gear for all body types and sizes or by offering customization for free, given the prices paid for quality outdoor gear. Mainstream outdoor media and industry should show representation of all marginalized folks while simultaneously giving back to these communities (by sponsoring camps and scholarships) so everybody knows they belong outdoors.

Outdoor community means inclusion, safety, celebration, and support. The most joyous times I've experienced are the hikes and events I've participated in with Fat Girls Hiking. Each occasion has given me the most incredible memories, which have led to special friendships and connections. Nothing tops the joy I feel when I'm enveloped by nature with these humans. I face personal challenges in the outdoors, even when I'm with a supportive community—the mental

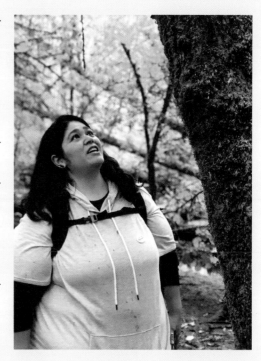

Ginamarie admires moss on a tree in Portland, Oregon

and emotional battle of feeling like I don't belong is hard, but I remind myself that hiking is not about speed, distance, or the finish, but rather the journey and surroundings.

Everyone belongs outdoors. I was terrified on my first hike, but taking that initial step changed my life in every way. If you can find support in family, friends, or a community you identify with, take them with you. If not, you can go solo—there is so much magic in being alone in nature. Start small, stay safe, bring snacks, let people know where you are, and breathe it all in.

GREENOUGH PARK
MISSOULA, MONTANA

Shelby (she/her)
FGH Chapter: Northern Montana

Being out in nature doesn't require me to defend or deny my size. I got grit and I got girth. The outdoors has helped me live in that largeness, and when I'm on the trail, I feel like my best self.

The mountain town of Missoula sits only four miles from the Rattlesnake Wilderness. Greenough Park is a gateway to this vast recreational corridor. There is little elevation gain, so these trails are perfect for any level.

DISTANCE ROUND TRIP Each loop is approximately half a mile.

ELEVATION GAIN 23 feet

CELL SERVICE Yes

ADA AND GENERAL ACCESSIBILITY The park includes two loops. The outer route is paved and wide enough to share with walkers, bikers, and anyone using mobility

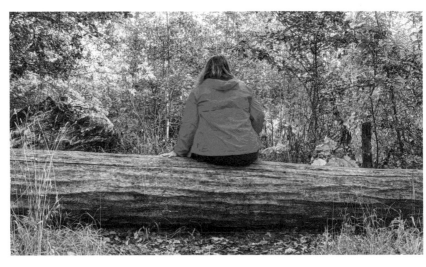

FGH NW Montana ambassador Shelby rests on a log

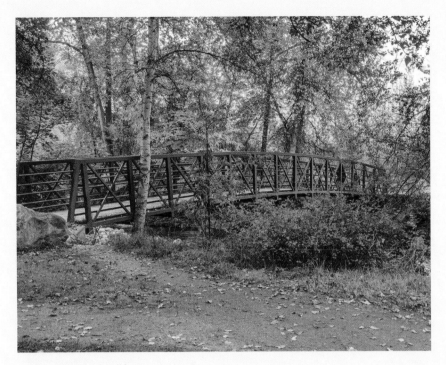

Bridge on the paved trail loop

aids or wheelchairs. The paved loop includes several bridges and views of the creek as it ribbons around shaded corners. The inner loop is dirt and more narrow—it's also closed to bikers.

BATHROOMS None

NATIVE LANDS Salish Kootenai

TRAIL DESCRIPTION The trails, maintained year round, loop around Rattlesnake Creek through a riparian forest. Both routes include benches, logs, and boulders for a contemplative rest. A favorite of birders and naturalists, the park is also visited by bear and moose. Dogs are allowed on leashes. If visiting in winter, be sure to bring appropriate footwear to navigate any icy patches.

OFFICIAL PARK ADDRESS Greenough Park, 1001 Monroe St, Missoula, MT 59802

TRAIL NAME Rattlesnake Creek Trail

HOW TO FIND THE TRAILHEAD The parking lot just north of Locust Street is where the paved route starts. If you'd like to begin on the dirt loop, drive just a little farther to the second parking lot near the covered picnic area on the left.

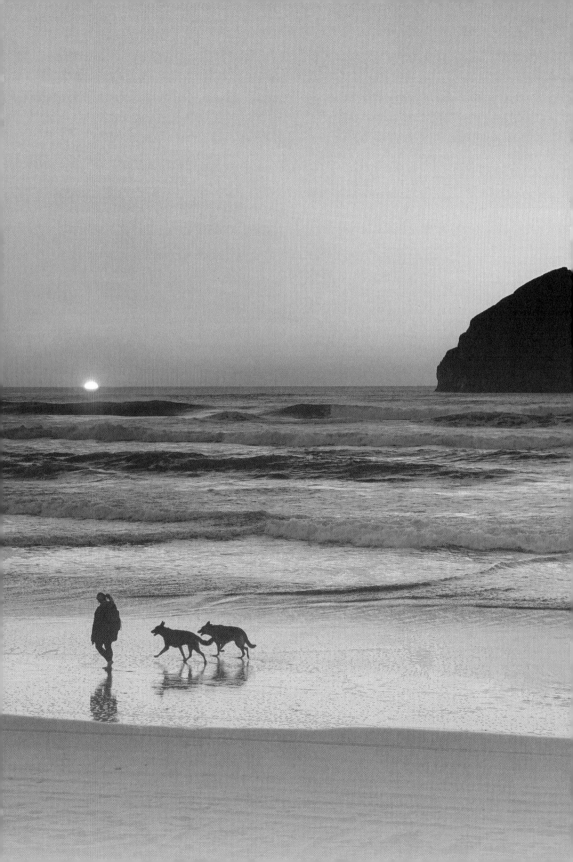

ACKNOWLEDGMENTS

I have wanted to write and publish a book since I was a teenager. It's a dream I never thought possible. Even with a writing degree and a lifetime of experience as a writer, it seemed unachievable. There are so many people who have fostered the creation of this book and supported me, the work I do in the outdoor industry, and the writing of this book.

First, I want to acknowledge Will McKay, the acquisition editor at Timber Press. From our first meeting at a coffee shop in downtown Portland, I felt like I really had someone rooting for my work. I had no idea how to write a book or how to make that writing into a manuscript. His support and answers to questions I had along the way fostered a space for me to create the book I dreamed of for Fat Girls Hiking. He believes in my voice, and that has been endlessly helpful throughout a very tumultuous year—2020 was not the year any of us thought it would be, but his patience and kindness and expert advice pushed me along when I wanted to give up. Thank you, Will!

Timber Press took a chance on me, an unpublished writer, and knew I had stories worth sharing. Thank you Timber Press for giving me the opportunity to share my writing and the stories of our community with the world.

The reality of writing a book while living in a van is not as glamorous as you might imagine. I lived in two kinda-broken-down vans before getting the van I have now. I didn't have a reliable home where I could feel safe and work until I got a message from Angela Lush on Instagram. I was

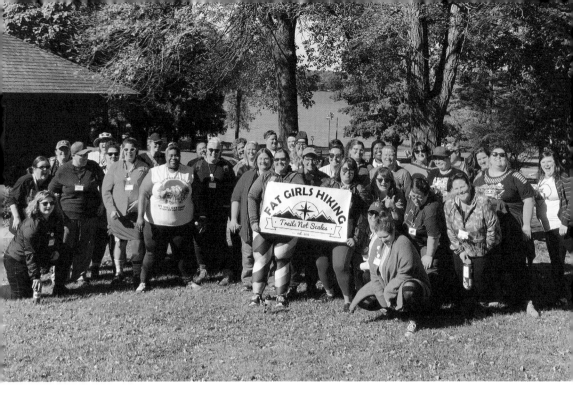

Radical Health Alliance organized Rad Fat Adventure Camp, a traditional camp experience with fat liberation at the center

looking for a new van to call home after my old one broke down, and she so generously offered the Sprinter van she had been traveling in for three years. She was going back home to Australia and would no longer need it. Thank you, Angela, for giving me a very good deal on the van and a very long payment plan. Without this incredible offer, I don't know that I would have been in a place mental-health wise, to write this book. To have a safe and reliable home on wheels vastly improved my well-being.

I also want to thank the people that have made the Oregon coast, which I now call home, into a place that fosters my creativity—together you gave me the space to keep writing. Kathy Jean, I am so grateful for you in my life. You support and love me and I am so glad to be your daughter. You introduced me to Lorie Welch, who offered me a safe place to park my van every night when a pandemic shut everything down and was terrorizing the world. Thank you, Lorie, for taking me in and letting me love this beautiful land you've made into such a healing place for me to write.

I feel so honored to be able to share the stories of many people in the FGH community with you. The community is the reason why I love my work. Thank you to every person who contributed time, photographs, and stories. You all are beautiful humans, and I am so grateful to know you.

The FGH ambassadors have created communities in their areas that foster safer outdoor spaces for marginalized folks. I am so thankful to each of you for being part of growing this community. Thank you to those that shared reviews of local trails. I appreciate the time, energy, and work you put into expanding this book.

To the people in my life who support me, cheer for me, and see my potential when I'm struggling: I could not have done this without you. Robin Heil-Kern, my mama, you gave me the gift of life. You put a camera

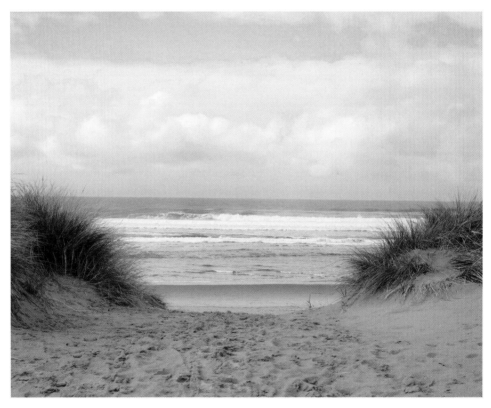

I'm forever grateful for the healing powers of the ocean

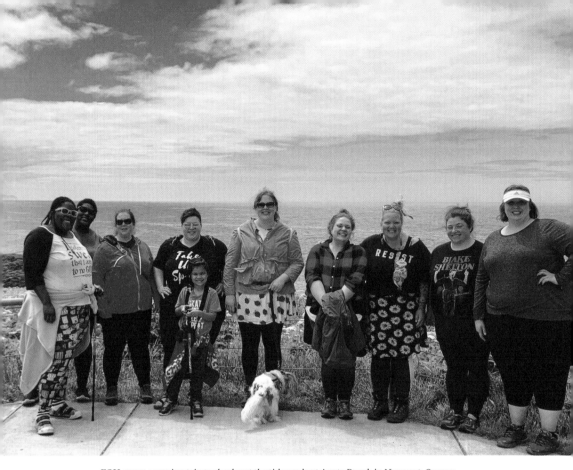

FGH group camping trip to check out the tide pools at Agate Beach in Newport, Oregon

in my hands, and I loved what I saw through the lens. Thank you for supporting me and my art and reminding me how precious and loved I am. I love you more than anything. Sarah Heil, my sister, you taught me so much when we were growing up and are always there for me when I need anything. Thank you! Thanks for creating one of my favorite humans, my niece, Veda. Veda, you give me hope for this world. You are an incredible leader and ally. I see the future of feminism, social justice, and joy when we talk. I love you!

To my besties, Ginamarie Simpson, Katie Danger Boone, and Sarah Hostetler, who came into my life through Fat Girls Hiking, thank you for listening, processing, and making me laugh when stuff feels rough. Thank you for reading my early writings for this book. Thank you for your feedback, ideas, and love. Ginamarie, you are my FGH partner, the Merch Queen, always coming up with new and fun ways to engage with the community. I appreciate all the work you do behind the scenes to keep the community, and me, going. Katie, thank you for so many great conversations over the years. And so many laughs! Your insight and perspective have always given me pause for thought. Sarah, you give support in so many ways. The ideas and comfort you bring to others in the community are so important. Thank you for leading hikes in the Portland area. I know this community is better with you in it.

The last acknowledgment I want to make is to the Fat Girls Hiking community. We have built this incredible space together. Thank you for being here. You matter.

RESOURCES

Whether you're looking for further reading, great social media accounts to follow, or online articles to expand your understanding of body liberation, fat activism, fat positivity, and outdoor recreation, check out these resources:

BOOKS

Things No One Will Tell Fat Girls: A Handbook for Unapologetic Living by Jes Baker

Landwhale: On Turning Insults Into Nicknames, Why Body Image Is Hard, and How Diets Can Kiss My Ass by Jes Baker

The Ultimate Guide to Plus-Size Backpacking: Travel Light. Whatever Your Size. by Edith Bernier

The Unapologetic Fat Girls Guide to Exercise and Other Incendiary Acts by Hanne Blank

Fat Activism: A Radical Social Movement by Charlotte Cooper

Hunger: A Memoir of (My) Body by Roxane Gay

What We Don't Talk About When We Talk About Fat by Aubrey Gordon

Big Fit Girl: Embrace the Body You Have by Louise Greene

Happy Fat: Taking Up Space in a World That Wants to Shrink You by Sofie Hagen

Lessons from the Fat-O-Sphere: Quit Dieting and Declare a Truce with Your Body by Kate Harding

Big Gal Yoga: Poses and Practices to Celebrate Your Body and Empower Your Life by Valerie Sagun

The Fat Studies Reader edited by Esther Rothblum and Sondra Solovay

Every Body Yoga: Let Go of Fear, Get on the Mat, Love Your Body by Jessamyn Stanley

Fearing the Black Body: The Racial Origins of Fat Phobia by Sabrina Strings

The Body is Not an Apology: The Power of Radical Self-Love by Sonya Renee Taylor

Celebrate Your Body (and Its Changes, Too!): The Ultimate Puberty Book for Girls by Sonya Renee Taylor

You Have the Right to Remain Fat by Virgie Tovar

A Beautiful Work in Progress by Mirna Valerio

Fat? So!: Because You Don't Have to Apologize for Your Size by Marilyn Wann

Shrill: Notes from a Loud Woman by Lindy West

ONLINE ARTICLES AND RESOURCES

"Everything You Know About Obesity is Wrong" by Michael Hobbes

Be Nourished blog and workshops (benourished.org)

The Body Is Not an Apology (thebodyisnotanapology.com)

The Militant Baker (themilitantbaker.com)

Your Fat Friend on *Medium* and yourfatfriend.com

INSTAGRAM

Art and Graphic Design

@alexisamannart

@artifats_collection

@csuggsillustration

@fat.designer

@frances_cannon

@joannathangiah

@kathrynhack

@littlearthlings

@mayakern

@mikalina

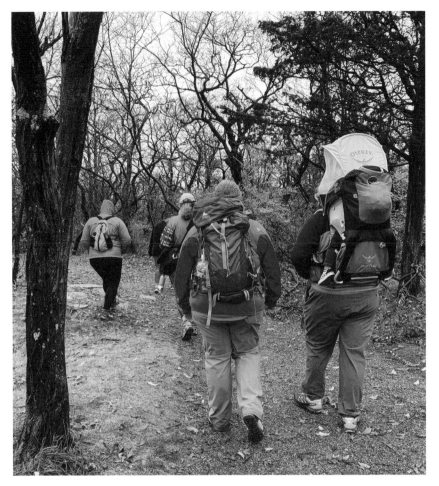

Hiking with an inclusive community boosts self confidence and offers a healing space for ourselves and others

@mollyccostello

@moosekleenex

@neoqlassicalart

@positevelypresent

@recipesforselflove

@shelby.bergen

@shoogsart

@sonialazo

@stephaniechinnart

@stinegreveillustration

@sugarygarbage

@yallaroza

@zaftig.art

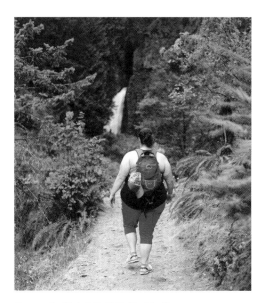

Amy on the Wahclella Falls Trail in Oregon

Photography

@bodyliberationwithlindley
@girlinwaterphotography
@historicalfatpeople
@kailawalton
@samortizphoto
@shooglet

Outdoors

@ashleysadventure
@brownpeoplecamping
@disablednoutdoors
@downwithadventure
@fatgirlforthefitsoul
@fattyonthefly
@feministbirdclub
@indigenouswomenhike

@latinooutdoors
@latinxhikers
@outdoorafro
@thefatgardener
@themirnavator
@vero_wandering

Movement

@louisegreen_bigfitgirl
@amberkarnesofficial
@theunderbellyyoga
@jabbieapp
@decolonizing_fitness
@kanoagreene
@chilltash
@radicalbodylove
@transyogateacher
@jessicajadeyoga

Communities

@fat.besties
@fatgirlstraveling
@fatwanderbabes
@fatwomenofcolor
@outdoorjournaltour

Fat Activism

@fat_baaaby
@fatlibink
@fatphobiaslayer
@thebodyisnotanapology
@thefatsextherapist
@yrfatfriend

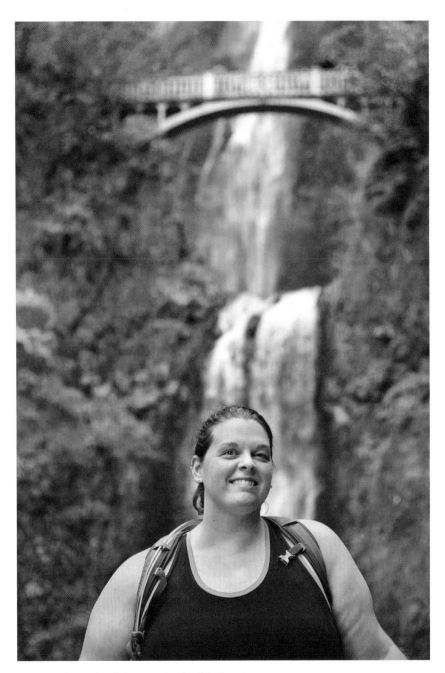

Amy at Multnomah Falls in Oregon's Columbia River Gorge

@alpinecurves
@cakeplussize
@copperunion
@fat.mermaids
@fatfancy
@fatgirlflow
@fatgirlflow
@proudmaryfashion
@stayfatdesignco
@superfithero

@chairbreaker
@femmebirds
@outtheadv
@plussizetransguy
@qpochikers
@queernature
@theventureoutproject

@benourishedpdx
@nalgonapositivitypride
@radicalhealthalliance

@diversifyvanlife
@doesthiscountasvanlife
@lonewolf.casita
@plusside_life
@thehappylands
@vanlifepride
@wander.free.and.queer
@whereistiffany

APPS

All Go
Big Fit Girl
Jabbie App
The Underbelly

PODCASTS

Maintenance Phase
Matter of Fat
Nomads at the Intersections
Out There
She Explores
She's All Fat
The Fat Lip
Trail Dames

FILMS

Fat Hiking Club
Fattitude

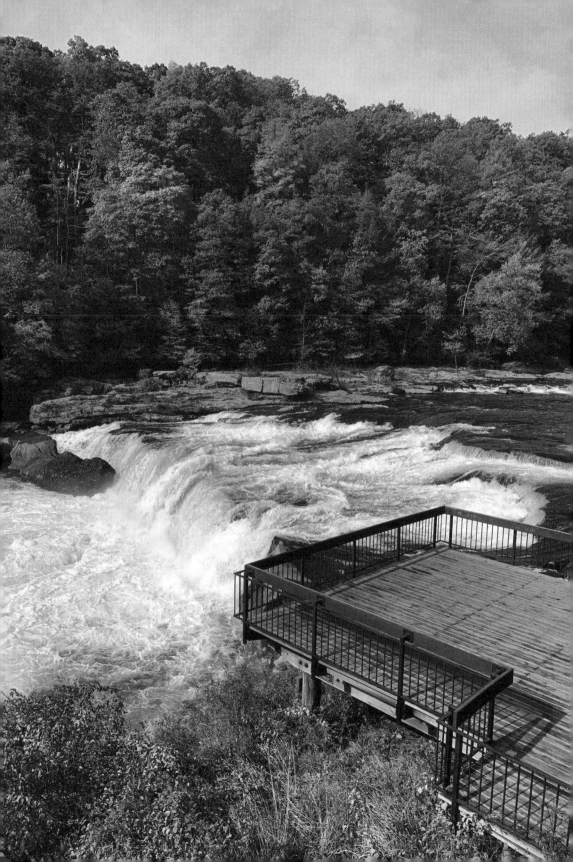

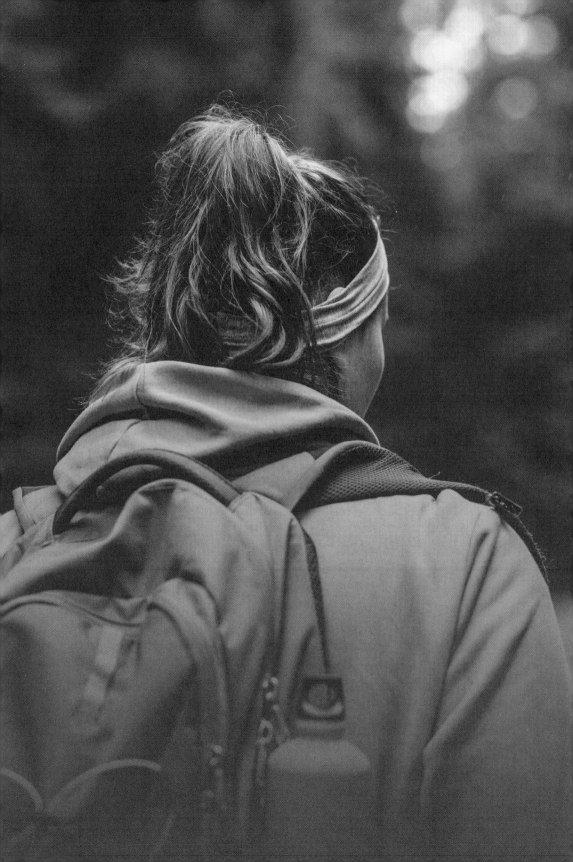

PHOTO CREDITS

INDEX

ABOUT THE AUTHOR

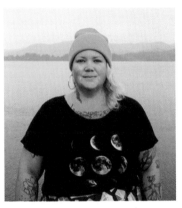

Summer Michaud-Skog is the founder of Fat Girls Hiking, a hiking community centered on a fat activism mission to get folks of diverse backgrounds out on trails no matter their size, ability, or experience level. With more than 35,000 Instagram followers, and thirty-six (and counting) official chapters across the world, FGH continues to grow by the day. "Trails Not Scales" is their motto, and it's all powered by Summer's grassroots efforts, tireless work ethic, and welcoming attitude. Summer also holds a degree in creative writing and is a photographer.